By the time you
Read this
I may be dead.
You cannot begin to comprehend
the thought of your death . . .
Until it becomes a real possibility!

Part one

One

My name is Peter and I'm sixty six years of age. I had cancer four and a half years ago and was treated with radiation after an operation to remove the lump from my neck. I left the cancer center thinking I would never return. But now here it is 2011 and I'm not too sure.

I woke up this morning the same time as I always do. Six thirty; lay there until seven then rise and dress. I walk down the two steps from the bedroom and go turn the propane stove on and set the coffee pot on it. I have my routine down pat. Next I raise the blinds and stare out across the lake and then I go outside and start the generator. Back inside I take two coffee cups out of the left hand cupboard and set them on the counter.

My biggest decision of the morning; have cereal and milk or ask Carol to make the big breakfast. Because today is probably going to be like all the rest I decide on cereal and milk. Apparently at my currant age I should be eating that healthy bran crap. At least that's what she says. I find it easier to go with the flow than defend myself and somehow I think it makes her feel like she's doing the right thing. After all she does know better than me. I must say here and now, I think I'm happy. How does one really know if he's happy or is in such a rut he makes himself believe he's happy? And what does it matter as long as everyone else thinks you're happy.

Some would have you believe this is a special week-end because it's the long week-end. Whoopee! To me it's just another week-end. Of course there are more campers here; all trying to convince themselves they must enjoy everything the long week-end has to offer. Don't get me wrong, they're all good people.

Today I will lie back in my lawn chair and once again wonder how long it will be before I get the call; the one I fear the most. Even the thought of the word biopsy makes me worry. Everyone says not to worry and of course I understand why they say it; what else can they say. Trust me; I worry because this is my second time to worry. I thought I had beaten it before but apparently I was wrong. I guess it's the waiting to find out for sure that really gets to me.

It makes me feel a bit better to hear the laughter of those around me. As I stare down the lake I think to myself, 'I will have to take six weeks or more out of my life again and go for treatment.' Don't ask me why but somehow I have it in my mind this time is going to be worse than the last time. I'm not a religious person but if I was at least I would have someone to blame. The best thing to do would be to suck it up and get ready for the big fight; easier said than done.

I look up to the crumbling clouds and let my mind wander. A Hummingbird hovers in the middle of my thoughts mere inches from my eyes. We have our understandings. I give them food and they in return give me many hours of entertainment. The clouds have their ways of forming that allow me a glimpse of pending doom. I see a half a devil's face peering out from behind a darker cloud . . . then it disappears.

My wife sits in her lawn chair doing her crosswords. I often wonder if she ever finds a new word after all these years of doing crosswords. I must remind myself to ask her some day. We are stagnant in our daily routines; yesterday, today and tomorrow, all the same.

I'd like to bring my canoe up to camp but why bother if I just have to take it back when I get the call. The breeze feels good on my face as the lake starts to come to life. Everyone here is safely caught up in their own doings. Me; my doings are yet to come. Of course once they stick the needle into that lump, I'll still have to wait yet again for how long is anyone's guess before they tell me what the next step is. I already know the next step; move the fifth wheel back into town so Carol can be more comfortable and get my mind set for what lie ahead.

The last time, I put on a brave face and made everyone except my wife believe that it was easy. It was not easy nor will it be this time. I think of my two children and four grand children and the great grandchild that's on the way. Somehow I manage to smile and for a brief moment remember what life is all about. I close my eyes and try to nap.

Black crows keep pecking at my dead body. I am helpless to move. I scream but no one hears me; no one comes to my rescue. I sit upright in my chair and realize that it was just a dream; perhaps a foretelling of the future! However there is a crow high up in a tree mocking me with its cawing. I must learn to dream healthier dreams.

Our silence is broken by the sound of a power boats racing towards the north. I think to myself, why so much power when this lake goes nowhere. Minutes after it passes the shore sounds out its complaints at the passing.

Tonight's campfire was interesting; at least eighteen campers sitting around it and chatting. For one couple it was their first fire of the season. You could see it by the way they stared into the flames. There were four young people roasting wieners also. Me, I just sat there contemplating life and watching everyone.

I went to bed at ten pm and went to sleep. I didn't talk to my wife again because I don't like to argue. You can't argue with silence. I hope tomorrow will make me feel better but I have my doubts.

Two

Today I rise at seven and put the coffee on. This mobius journey that I am on leads me through each day; waiting and wondering; yesterday, today and tomorrow all the same. Today is no different than all the others. Other than the morning clouds overhead I see no signs of change. I will sit in my lawn chair once again and stare down the lake and think of death.
On days like this when I'm doused in grey and I fear I'll not see the sun;
I wish I could just secret myself away until this dreary day be done.

No mountain tops can be seen through the clouds, there's only a lone sea gull high on the wing. Today I do not know what thoughts will be allowed, it is a most worrisome and troubling thing.

I sit here waiting for heavens down pouring with no hope of seeing the sun; off in the distance thunder is roaring. Oh why can't this dreary day be done? Sad poems are all that come out of me now. Melancholy

labours deep in my heart where I keep all my secrets. I sit
in this lawn chair waiting for the call.

Even the breeze seems to be mocking me . . . .
Damn! (My computer just crashed) my last five minutes
of thinking and writing is gone; gone and forgotten. I'm
sure it wasn't that important. Now . . . where was I?

As much as I try to think other thoughts all too often
it does not work. There are no delusions with my tears
though my thoughts are heavy like stone. There is the
fretting and the fear for I do not want to die alone.

I rise from my lawn chair and walk away from
everyone; not to be alone especially, just to be away
from them. A solitary loon just off shore distracts me for
the briefest moment. I think of his freedom. I sit down
with my feet dangling over the edge of the road and start
my thinking again. There is two of me. Sometimes I wear
myself inside out; sometimes not.

Tomorrow is already inside of me. Tonight I will
morph with the moon and become that other me. Ah
darkness; that secret agent of death that will torment me
when I'm gone. Sometimes when I awaken from that
other gentler death; my head full of bad dreams, I realize
there are two of me. Sometimes I don't like the other me.
Often we fight. Neither ever wins. I speak softly to the

loon as he dives silently beneath the water. He takes my thoughts with him.

There must be something I can do to alter this state of constant wondering. I tried yesterday when I went fishing with Gary. But all we did was talk about our problems. I know I'm not the only one. I guess life is just a problem we all must solve before . . . before you know?

I made a tee time for tomorrow. That's probably when I'll have to start communicating with Carol. I don't know if I'm madder at her for always arguing or me for always putting up with it. After all, what should I expect after forty three years? Maybe I'll just roll over and play dead. I'm sure life frustrates her sometimes too. I'd like to discuss it sometime when just the two of us are alone, but we seldom have meaningful conversations anymore; probably my fault.

I love golfing. I think the frustration of hitting a stupid little white ball correctly brings a person down to earth. I do understand the important things in life. I wish I could swing at death the way I do with my driver. Maybe that's exactly what I am doing! I'll have to ponder that tonight around the campfire.

Last night I laid my head upon my pillow and dreamed a dark and dreary poem. Ominous words heavy with sleep oozing into the darkness of my soul. I do not dream of death often.

My eyes wander to the trees across the lake and I think; I am like the forest, some of my scars run deep. She has her hidden secrets and I have a few I must keep. I am like the forest. I have my quiet moods. I too will carry on with my many interludes.

It's starting to rain so go inside to watch the hockey game. I'm so not a Vancouver Canuck fan but my sister and brother in law are. They have no television. I do love their company so that's fine with me. We sit and chat about nothing. The sound of the rain on our slide out is soothing.

Tomorrow is a holiday so I will not get the call then; maybe the day after. Why do people tell you to be patient when it's not them who are anxious? It seems to be my daily chore to just sit here and endure time. I ponder the intent of time that my course would steal, and flee. This moment, now is the only thing I relish in this suspended destiny.

Today the rain never stopped. It pounded at my thoughts well into the night. No campfire for anyone.

Fired the generator up and watched the boob tube. My next big question is when should I go to bed? The darkness makes me think of death; and the quietness gets inside of me and troubles my dreaming. Tomorrow I will bolster my spirit with positive thinking. Yes, that is what I will do.

Three

Today it's the same old, same old. My first thought of the day; when will I get the call? I must prepare myself for the worst. Radiation leaves little or no visible scars. Emotional scars; now that's another thing altogether. I try to avoid some of the other campers because they only compound my anxiety with their words of wisdom. I guess we're all burdened with our human frailties. Stiff upper lip and all that stuff is all any of them can think to say. I am learning how to wait; silence ribbons through me as I contemplate a happier tomorrow.

Tonight the sky has opened the clouds to reveal a magnificent bright sky. The night-sky is sifting her universal tints from heaven's high glittering sieve. She shakes the remains of her embers where in glittering silence she lives. I witness a fire-glow in the trembling womb of night, an ecstasy of incandescent burning. The brightness of her shattered light sets this mortal heart to yearning.

Yesterday, today and tomorrow march by one by one taking me to my uncertain future. I sit, I wait and I ponder. I might as well come right out and say it; speak that word that has teetered on the tip of my thinking. "Cancer" one word says it all. The strange thing is I try to justify that I am glad it is me that has it rather than one of my loved ones. What kind of a bizarre thought is that?

Don't get me wrong I am glad I am the only one in my family that has it.

Alcohol does seem to help numb the senses and boost my resolve to fight it. I have thoughts of suicide every now and then; not actually doing myself in; more like weighing all the options should a depressing decision have to be made. One must be ready you know. I think of the suicide note and what it should say. Maybe something like; I have reached the no more of me and it is now time to concede to this battle that is taking its victory. Yes that would be dignified and to the point. Of course that would only happen as a last resort. I'm not a coward; not yet anyway. I'll just have to wait and see what metal I'm made of. It is my great worry I will fold like a cheap lawn chair when the going gets tough. You'll be the last to know by the way. My exterior is still rock solid and impenetrable.

My father died of Cancer and my step father also. I know if I had the courage that my late mother had I could fight it with one hand tied behind my back. But alas, I am me and must accept what I am dealt. This is my therapy of a sort; this splashing of my words onto this page. Today I abandon my thoughts on this page; these words drawn from the grim depths of my soul. I bare the whole of it, you none.

I consider myself a writer. There are those who would disagree with that statement. I guess the proof is in the pudding; so to speak. I know sesquipedalian words. Of course the word, "sesquipedalian is a polysyllabic word; but you already knew that!

These words are my filter between the hard reality of today and the pending uncertainties of tomorrow. Brave words can be conjured up to fortify my spirit. I will fight the fight and will never cease in my endeavour.

Today has given me permission to carry on; I have been reprieved. Oh sure I still have my boundaries. I do not believe what I once believed. I now use more cautionary discretion. This waiting has changed me . . . inside. But for now today keeps me centered and holds me to this endeavor. I must never, say never. This day has given its full consent; it is a sort of delayed execution. What is finally decided will be my ultimate fate. Maybe tomorrow I will get the call.

No; not today. Damn this relentless assault on my senses. Who do they think I am that I can sit here without worry or care? I suspect my cancer knows and feeds off my fret. I reach up and feel the lump yet again, trying to will it away. Will the needle hurt when it is shoved into it? The answer is yes; it sure as hell hurt the other time. And now I know it will hurt it's probably going to hurt even more. God, I'm such a sissy; Thank God no one knows for sure, except me. I try to lock the thought up inside of me and not think about it. It does no good.

Today we golf. Ah that freedom to release all that pent up unknowing in me. "There, take that" I say as I smash the ball two hundred and thirty three yards down the left side of the fairway. Now it's just me and this stupid game. As I size up my next shot to the green I realize life is like a game of golf; No matter how hard we try to avoid the traps we often fail. It's how we get out of those traps that define us as a person. We all have our handicaps and how we handle them determines where we go from there. Some simply accept their misfortunes and think of them as failures. We all strive to make it to the nineteenth hole without too much misfortune. I wonder if my "nineteenth hole" will be another golf course or six feet under. Ones perspective in life like golf is what we make of it. Just in case you're interested I golfed rather poorly. But I did enjoy the company.

It worked; Carol and I are talking again. It's always easier to reflect on your troubles after they have faded into the background. I don't want to get mad at her for arguing over the most trivial of thing but sometimes it just gets to me. I will work harder at trying to ignore the petty things and concentrate on the good things; like where would I be without her. That thought scares me. She has many other endearing qualities.

I know tomorrow will be the day I get the call. It has to be. If it is I'm ready to go. Of course after they do the biopsy there will be another round of waiting; waiting for the results, waiting for the next call as to when and where the treatment will be given. Yesterday, today and tomorrow will begin all over again.

Four

I don't know what to tell you now. It's been another three days and still no call. Is it only me that seems to think of this dilemma as an emergency? I guess when you think about it I am the only one that has the greatest investment it what the outcome will be.

Maybe it's time to think about God! No, I've done that in the past and it didn't work out then either. It was when I was ten years old and my father was dying of stomach cancer. My grandmother told me if I prayed really hard my dad would make it. I prayed as hard as any ten year old boy was capable of doing and my dad died; in spite of what my grandmother had said. I never blamed her for telling me that; I blamed God. Of course now in hindsight that was a ridiculous assumption. It only stand to reason if there was a God then my father never would have gotten cancer in the first place; just another one of life's traps.

Maybe it's my expectations that are part of my problem. I know I've always been a pessimist. Could be it's time I gave optimism a whirl; easier said than done of course. I'll buy a book and give it all I've got. I have given some thought to having no expectations whatsoever. But how does one set their mind on that course and keep it there. I would think it is probably impossible. I once heard it said that disappointments are life's tiny testers; you could either let them take you down or use them to build yourself back up. Good sound advice if you ask me.

I'm not too sure the thought of having cancer qualifies as one of life's "little testers." I'm almost certain it has nothing to do with any test. Of course when you think about it, it is not something I brought on myself. I didn't rob a bank and now must deal with the disappointment of my decisions. No, I am disappointed that I have no choice in the cause of my problem but must find a solution to beat it. Perhaps disappointment is the wrong word to use. I feel better when I say I'm frustrated and pissed off.

I have given some thought to the possibility I'm just wasting your time and mine by even writing this. What if my cancer isn't back? Is this just another squandering of my time and yours? Perhaps not; we can both learn from what goes on in the mind when we are faced with life changing dilemmas. It helps me when I write things down. I find it's a great release for my woes.

We were making a list of things we needed when we go to town. I emptied the Yuban coffee can into our other coffee container and said to myself, "Good, I can use this can."

Carol looked up from her crossword book and said, "You can't make a toaster out of that can because it's made of cardboard."

Now let me ask you this . . . how big a moron does she think a person would be to make a toaster to use over a propane flame that was made out of cardboard? It took every ounce of my will to keep my mouth shut and not blow up again. Sometimes I wonder if she even realizes what she says. I hope not. It did occur to me to seriously tell her I could make a toaster out of it; it's just I could only use it once. I'm learning to bit my tongue more and more. I think that's what most men have to do to keep their marriages going. I had another purpose for the coffee can in mind and will use it for that. I'll just keep looking for one that can be used to make a toaster.

Today I'm driving her into town so she can golf her first ladies day of the year. This will be the first day I'll have for myself in over eight months. I must tell you I am looking forward to it. I'll probably get to work on my next novel. I'm dwelling less and less on when I'll get the call. I think it will come in the next few days and I'm ready.

I just remembered I had a dream last night. I'm sure it was about death. I was standing at the top of a bunch of wide steps looking down. At the bottom there was a monstrous bull with great big horns and he was looking up at me and snorting. I wasn't afraid but somehow I knew it was death. The bull started running up the steps as I calmly stood there waiting. When he reached the top I put both hands out to meet him and shoved him back down the steps. There was no panic whatsoever while this was happening.

The bull tumbled end over end and landed at the bottom and charged again. This time he came faster and more determined. I held my ground and pushed him backwards with all my strength. He tumbled to the bottom and charged again. I ran ten feet to my left where there were more steps that went down to the landing where the bull had come from. It chased me up and down the steps until I woke up. I think it means I can avoid death for a certain length of time but it is going to tire me out and get me in the end. I can tell you this though, it was one of the most vivid dreams I've ever had. Of course it may just have been a dream that meant nothing at all. I guess it's what you make of it.

Five

The last time I had cancer I found myself crying more often than what should be normal. Carol says its normal; I beg to differ. The first time when I had cancer and I was driving down to the cancer center I started thinking what a lucky person I was in spite of cancer. I had the finest woman for a wife any man could have. I knew I didn't deserve to have her love and support. I thought about how I'd failed her over the years, especially in retirement. She certainly deserved better than me. Then I started thinking about our two children and how happy they were in their marriages and the two grand-children they each had. Once again I started to cry; for no apparent reason I could not hold back the tears. I pulled to the side of the highway and composed myself for the rest of the trip. Again, as I write this I fight the tears. I hope they're tears of joy. It seems I cry far too much. Cancer did that to me; that's the only explanation I can come up with.

One would think if you have to go through a second treatment it would be easier; one would think. So far with me it is not easier, if anything the waiting is far more stressful this time. I think that is because the last time my surgeon said not to worry because it probably wasn't cancer.

That time when he phoned me and told me it was, I couldn't speak. I wrote the name Acinar Cell Carcinoma on a piece of paper in front of me. When I got off the phone my wife asked me what the doctor had just said and I could not speak. I pointed to the piece of paper and went to our bedroom and wept like a baby; I didn't want to but I felt so helpless. Up until that phone call we had never said the word. But we sure as hell heard it a lot after that. Acinar Cell Carcinoma; I'd never heard of it before. I'll never forget his words; "It's a rare as shit from a rocking horse." Apparently he thought that was funny. I did not think it was funny.

My saving grace was the people that helped me through the process. I can't praise the staff at the cancer center enough. It must be hard on them having to deal with this sort of thing day in and day out. I don't know how they manage to keep their positive attitudes all the time. Whatever they're getting paid it is probably not enough.

I just hope I get the chance to look back on all of this. I wonder what my perspective will be then. I'll probably wonder why I worried in the first place. Looking back is what I must look forward to. I think it was Helen Keller who once said, "We could never learn to be brave and

patient if there were only joy in our lives." Can't argue
with that philosophy can you?

Today I'm starting to write another novel. Writing
takes my mind off things and keeps me safe from the
turmoil of unwanted thoughts. Once my mind zeros in on
what I'm writing I get lost in time. Nothing can deter me
until I run out of words. I can only write poetry when I'm
alone; that's why I don't write when Carol's here.

Poetry is my bench that sags under the weight of
my thoughts. I feel its simple structure about me and am
sheltered with the strength and the protection it offers.
It's a bed for my soul; that receptacle that becomes
either a lounge of comfortability or a place to hide from
the reality of truth.

There is no place I'd rather be than where I am
today. I sit here happy and carefree with the whole day
to while away. I sit and listen to nature's sounds and
admire the clouds floating by. No more serenity have I
ever found; I truly am a contented guy.

Tonight when Carol returns from golf with her sister
I'll have the barbeque hot and ready to cook her supper.
I'll listen intently while she tells me about how her day
went. We'll have a campfire and I'll stare into the flames

and wonder, will I get the call tomorrow? Tomorrow will come; eventually.

I wish I could be completely alone all the time or at least until all this is behind me; one way or the other. But I know it would be selfish of me to attempt something so daring as that. But just the same if I had my druthers I definitely would like to be by myself for the next couple of months. I wouldn't have the chutzpah to approach Carol about that one. She thinks I need her and everyone one else around me, and sometimes I suppose I do. But the way I feel right now; this very minute, I really would like to be alone.

A fellow camper by the name of Rienk Rienks just came over while there was no one around and told me if I need to be driven any where he will gladly do it. I understand how generous an offer that is and know he is sincere about it. But I do not want to be beholding to anyone unless I have to. I thanked him for his generosity and told him I was going to make my decisions when they have to be made.

Now, where was I; oh yeah, I'm enjoying my time by myself. The sky has filled with clouds. I hope it does not rain at the golf course. The silence here along the lake is splendidly pleasant. It's so quiet I can almost hear my thoughts; thoughts that lead me to my task of writing. I think of words as though they are my own personal arsenal. I can hurl them at my distracters. I possess a battery of words; black thick words oozing night; radiant words bringing light; bold confident words marching in rows like soldiers smartly on duty. Explosions of expression blasted onto this white plain of indifference before me; wicked words festering in the wound of humiliation and shame; soft words pure and puffy and fluffy, and heavy words sinking into the sunset; pulling day under. I also have transparent words that I can weave into the gossamer dreams at my waking. But again they are only words.

    I had mild Italian sausages barbequed for supper. Damn they tasted good. I'll do the other two when Carol gets home from golf. Who knows, it might be to my advantage to make supper for her. I'll just have to wait and see. I started the campfire at six hoping the girls would like to sit around it when they got back. It turns out that Dawn and Gary wanted to watch the hockey game and as it was raining a bit Carol only came to the fire for one drink. That left me alone for the next three hours while they watched hockey. I did a lot of deep thinking; looking into the flames does that to me. I came to the conclusion that I've been too negative lately. That probably has something to do with depression. I think I'm making progress in trying to figure things out. I was ready for a fight when I came inside but I was surprised at how well I handled it. All in all it was a great day. But you already knew that.

Six

I slept soundly last night. I woke this morning to the sound of rain on our roof. I had hoped to golf today but that doesn't look like it will happen. I don't like staying inside all day long. It gives me too much time to think about discouraging things. Maybe we'll go into town and see what happens. Carol is still sleeping. I hope she had a good night's rest. If I want to check my cell phone messages I have to drive fifteen mile towards town until I pick up a signal. I really am expecting the call today.

A thought just occurred to me; what if somehow they forgot about me. What if they lost my file? How long should I wait until I call my doctor again? I think now I'm getting paranoid. It's hard enough waiting never mind waiting on a sombre grey rainy day. It seems to me every morning when I get out of bed I have to start all over at bringing my spirits up.

I must make a point of being extra tentative to Carol this morning. It might take my mind of everything else. Maybe I should learn how to control my mind better. I probably don't have enough time to accomplish any degree of success before . . . you know. Today I will focus on happy thoughts and pleasant things. I know; I'll think about my great granddaughter that is due in eight weeks. That shouldn't be too hard.

There, I feel much better. Now let's get on with the day. Carol says she doesn't want to golf today because she thinks it's too wet; so that's that.

I should go to where I can get cell service; otherwise it's going to weigh on my mind all day. As much as I don't want to drive that far I know I will so I might as well get on with it. I'll be back within the hour.

I just got back and there were no messages on my phone. Maybe I'm the only one who cares. I did go to town and get the paper for Carol. On the way back I thought about stopping at the last place I can get cell service and wait until the damn thing rings.

Another thing I noticed was what the highways department is doing about their potholes. It's quite ingenious when you think of it. They're letting them get so big you can spot them from a quarter of a mile away, thus allowing you to drive around them. Who would have thought? We could have golfed as the weather in town was okay.

I just received an e-mail from my older sister in Calgary; the one with the broken foot. She tells me she's trying to get a ride out here with a friend of hers. In a way I hope she does and in another way I'm not so sure. It's hard when too many people start telling you to keep a stiff upper lip. But it would be nice to visit with her; we'll see.

Today there's just me and Carol in camp and it's nice and peaceful. She does her crosswords and I do this. I have my doubts about seeing the sun at all today. I was wrong. The sun just peeked out and I'm out the door. See you later.

Carol joined me and we sat and talked. When I told her a friend had offered to drive me anywhere should I have to go for treatment I choked up and could hardly get the words out. Like I told you earlier, I cry far too easily now. At least I talked to her about it.

We had chicken quesadillas for supper; my favorite. Sometimes I can be such a glutton. Carol wanted to watch American idol because it was the two hour grand finale. I didn't so I went and lit the campfire and sat there by myself. For some reason I started reflecting back on my childhood. My mind went back to the time I was eight years old and my father, who was a giant of a man ordered me to go down to the barn in the dark and get the pitch fork because our dog had treed a cougar behind our house and he was out of ammunition.

Even though I was a skinny kid I looked at my father and said, "No way, I ain't going out of the house." Now, I knew what the strap felt like and I didn't care at that moment. If you think I'm going out that front door and there's a cougar behind the house . . . I don't think so; bring the strap on. He must have seen the resolve in my eyes because he went and got it himself. While he was gone I thought to myself, "What good is a pitch fork against a cougar that's probably thirty or forty feet up a tree." Maybe he was going to impale it with an accurate throw. I haven't thought about that incident for many years.

What does it mean? Am I getting everything in order? I left the campfire after that reminiscence. I didn't want to see what the next one was going to be. It's raining out now so that suits me just fine. I'll go to bed and listen to it on our slide-out. Tomorrow I think we are going golfing.

When I went out to start the generator this morning I noticed the wind was coming out of the north and it was quite warm. The nights are getting warmer too. We still can't sit outside and enjoy our coffees in the morning just yet. I didn't want to get out of bed this morning. Sometimes when I'm holding Carol I just want to stay in the comfort of the moment. I haven't told her I love her in a long time. Maybe today would be a good day to do that. I do love her and I'm sure she knows it. Mind you, she hasn't told me those words in a long time either. I guess after forty five years together we just get in a rut. Maybe I should get her a single red rose like I used to do when the kids were growing up. It was to let her know how much I appreciated her and loved her. But I suppose if I give her one now she'll think I'm apologizing for something. Of course I could just give her one and let her think whatever she wants.

    I remember a poem I wrote to her many long years ago.

    When a beautiful woman begins to smile and upon you applies her folly, surrender to that deceptive guile that would ease your melancholy.

    Today when we got back from golfing in the rain there was a message in my e-mail from my daughter in law telling me to phone the doctor on Monday to make an appointment for the biopsy. Now at least I'm getting closer to having it done. I'll have to wait for another three days before I can phone. I wonder how long I'll have to wait after the appointment is made. I'm sure there are

many unfortunate people out there worse off than me.
There's always someone worse off than me.

Carol's making rhubarb crisp this afternoon. We
bought ice cream to go with it. Is there anything more
comforting than hot rhubarb crisp with vanilla ice cream?
Not for me there isn't. My mouth is salivating as I write.

Seven

I woke to rain once again this morning. I know I'm supposed to wait until Monday to phone for my appointment but I'm going to town today and see if I can get it done. At least that way maybe I'll have a worry free weekend; maybe not. I've been on the internet lately looking for information that will help me deal with my anxiety. I found nothing that I hadn't discover the last time I had cancer. I wish I was the kind of person that could just sit down with someone and discuss it but I'm not and that is that. As strange as it may seem I do try to think of the most horrific things that have happened around the world and then hope I will feel better about my problem. That doesn't work and I was stupid to even think it would.

I feel the helpless frustration building in me now. I want to do something; anything. Today and tomorrow are not going to be good days. I hope we don't have any visitors today because I definitely do not want to talk meaningless trivia.

Did you ever notice how little some people actually have to say? If you could eliminate the weather and the gossip from a conversation most people would sit there dumb as a post with nothing to say. I would prefer that to the constant drivel that I am subjected to most of the time. And more times than not someone wants to tell you the same thing they told you yesterday; and probably will tell you tomorrow.

It's not that bad around the campfire though, no, most of the time someone will inject a bit of humor into the conversation and get people laughing. I like to focus on one individual and try to make them laugh. It loosens everyone up and gets them into the right mood. Of course sometimes it backfires when that person thinks I'm making fun of them in front of everyone. At times like that only quick thinking can save me from humiliation and staring eyes; especially my wife's. If I've had a few drinks, which most often is the case, I have been heard to say some rather crude things. Mustn't hurt any ones delicate feelings now must we?

That's another thing; some people are so damn sensitive. The other night I told a "fat joke" Two of the rather robust ladies at the fire never laughed at all. They just smoothed out their blankets that were coving their large frames and looked at each other. I must learn to be more sensitive; the way I see it, if you can't have a good chuckle around the campfire then where in the hell can you?

We're going to town in fifteen minutes to make that phone call. I'll let you know how it went when I get back.

.... I am so PISSED OFF right now. Stand back people, I'm about to blow. I phoned the doctor in Salmon Arm and got a voice message. There's something wrong about that; a voice message in a doctor's office, give me a break. No one will be in the office until 8:00 AM on Monday morning. Isn't that just great? I'll just sit here for two and a half days and twiddle my thumbs. I hope my exasperation doesn't cultivate an argument between me and Carol. I can't even go outside because the rain hasn't let up for so long.

The only good thing to come out of my call was at least now I know it is the same doctor that did the surgery the last time. I'm grateful for that as he is a great surgeon. I trust him completely. If you'll excuse me I'm going to go for a walk and try to calm down.

We just finished the last of the Rhubarb Crisp and it was the best I've ever had. It seems to me Carol is making a lot of great things to eat lately. Maybe she's trying to fatten me up. She probably remembers how much weight I lost from the radiation treatment the last time. Mind you she's always been a mighty fine cook; I'm already overweight now.

I woke to the sight of no rain today; had pancakes and sausages for breakfast. After that I went out and lay back in my lawn chair and looked up at a dull grey sky. A flock of sixty two geese flew northward over me. One side of the V was twice as long as the other. Do you know why that is? The answer might surprise you. A few years ago I had the pleasure to talk to a very old Indian chap by the name of Walter and he told me why that is. He said the reason one side of the V is longer is because there are more geese on that side. Stupid me here I was expecting some profound wisdom from an old man and what did I get . . . humor!

Carol wanted to vacuum this morning so I put the generator on. I had to put it to high throttle for the vacuum cleaner to work properly. When she finished I was going to put it back to normal throttle before I shut it down. She just came out side and turned it off. Of course that is hard on the generator. When I told her she should have put it back to normal throttle before she turned it off she took no responsibility for her actions. Her answer was, "I didn't know, you never told me."

What she should have said was, "Oh, I guess I should have asked before I did anything." I bit my tongue and stewed for a while and forgot about it. If I would have said what I normally would have said we wouldn't have spoken to each other for days. I guess that is what I must do from now on, even though I feel like it's giving in. If I'm going to give in then I might as well give up.

A half an hour ago I was on the computer and Carol was standing beside me. I said, "I'd like you to see this gadget that I down loaded that will help you search the internet easier."

She ignored everything I said. When she realized she had ignored me she came closer and started to ask what I had said. I simply threw my hands up in the air and went outside and sat in my lawn chair. I started thinking; why am I getting upset over her ignoring me? After all, who the hell do I think I am? It's not like it's the first time it's ever happened. It'll take me a while but I'll put it behind me just like all the other times she does thoughtless things.

Tonight we sat around the fire pit and it rained again. We all had umbrellas and toughed it out. It turned out to be a great night. And just for the record I did put her ignoring me behind me; but I haven't forgotten it.

Eight

What a pleasant surprise when I woke this morning to see the sunshine. I have only one more day until I phone my doctor. Today I will have a positive attitude.

I made a toaster for our propane stove top this morning. Yip! You guessed it; I made it out of a "TIN" coffee can. It's a damn fine looking toaster if you ask me. And I only cut myself three times. Those tin snips are hard to use on a round piece of metal. Of course when I was done I had to go around and show it off to anyone that was present. Carol says we should put it on the bonfire tonight to burn any harmful stuff off of it. Who am I to argue with that?

Now I'm looking for something else to keep my mind busy. Let me see . . .

When we had our campfire tonight Carol thought it would be a good idea to put the new toaster over the fire to burn the newness out of it. I thought that was a great idea so that's what we did. When she was satisfied it had seasoned enough I took it off and went to set it down to cool. Now here's the chuckle of the day. She said, and I repeat word for word; "Don't set it on the picnic table because it's hot. Of course our picnic table has a plastic table cloth on it. Now let me ask you this . . . how big a moron does she think a person would be to set a hot toaster on a plastic topped picnic table? I didn't know what to say. But all in all it really was a great day.

Wouldn't you know it, today I woke at five thirty? That tells me I'm eager to find out when my appointment is going to be. I wonder how long I'll have to wait for that. I'm not going to let it wreck my golf game today. If you can't be happy on the sunny days then when can you?
Here it is eight twenty already and we haven't left for town yet. For over two weeks I've been chomping at the bit to get things going and now I find myself unhurried. Don't ask me why that is. We're heading to town to make the call and golf. Wish me well!

I just got back from town. I have some good news and bad news. The good news is I got an appointment to see the doctor in Salmon Arm. The bad news is it's not for the biopsy. Apparently he has to see me and assess me first. It won't be for another nine days until I see him and God knows how long before they get around to doing the friggen biopsy.

Here we go again with the waiting. Not only that, I never golfed very well. Some days you just can't win. It seems to me I spend all my time trying to stay on an even keel. Tonight I'm going to bed with a positive attitude and a good woman by my side.

Guess what! We never went to bed together tonight. She decided to criticize the shorts I was wearing. I wear ratty shorts in camp and I have for a while ... We're in camp for #%$#%$# sakes!!!!! What's the big deal? I think she has this great need to criticize me. I must be a big pig and such a disappointment to her. I'll get her to pick my clothes out the night before so I'll be dressed to her liking. We wouldn't want me to look too unsightly in camp now would we?

She's golfing later today so maybe I'll wear whatever I like and hope the other two people around here don't snitch on me. We'll see. Now we're not talking to each other again. I don't know what to do anymore. If I could just find a way to ignore it every time she puts me down I would. But I really don't think patronizing someone is the answer. When I pick her up tonight I'll try my best to talk to her. If that doesn't work then I guess I'll start making plans to get this cancer thing over with and then maybe go out to the Island and visit my Brother. Everything always hangs on this cancer thing.

I will say it is nice and peaceful in camp today as I'm the only one here. This is the time when I can concentrate and write a poem.

Today I know not what my heart will allow; what singing breeze will dance out of this sunny unfolding.

Ah Breeze!
Ah! Breeze, whisper to me with your airy mood;
Bring out all this day's delightful passion.
If you were any more subdued you'd have nothing less to ration.
Ah! Breeze, with your soft flutter;
There's something about something fresh and new.
You cause the human heart to shutter just thinking about the magnificence of you.

There, that went well I think. Now I feel much better. Now it's time to lie back in the lawn chair and catch a few zzzz's. Who knows, maybe I'll have a pleasant dream.

I never dreamt at all but I did think about how angry I get sometimes. Maybe I'm directing my anger in the wrong direction. I know it's not on purpose if I am.

Maybe I get too angry at Carol because of my frustration over this damn cancer thing. I should let her know . . . she probably has already figured that out though.

When one of the other campers got back from town he asked me when my appointment for the biopsy was. When I told him I had to see the specialist first he said, "That's what makes me mad, everybody having to wait. Those doctors are just using the system."

I was shocked at his words. We don't know how the system works. It's probably not the doctor's fault at all. If anything we could blame the government. After all don't we blame them for everything we don't understand? I'm sure there are a lot of people out there worse off than me and they're probably more anxious. I can't blame anyone for something I know nothing about. I'm sure there are those who would say, "How long does he expect to live anyway?"

I'd like to answer those people. "I want to live just as long as you want to live. So you let me know how long you'd like to live." My only fear is it will drag on so long we won't be able to go to Arizona for the winter. That is not what I want.

Nine

I went to town today to see my dental hygienist and get my teeth cleaned. I know if I need radiation I must have my teeth up to par, and they are. After that I went for Chinese food. When I paid the waitress she handed me a fortune cookie so I opened it up and read the message. It said you will have the answer to your problem soon. Now that is good news isn't it? I'd like to believe that but I am a pessimist.

I spent the whole afternoon thinking again. The more I do it the more I am coming to realize it is not a good thing. My mood is the lowest it's been in over a month. I know I'm depressed and there is nothing I can do about it. I do take solace in my poetry, so I write what I am feeling.

There is a black hole in my spirit today that I somehow must once again endure.
I fear it might be here to stay for I have yet to discover the cure.
This hopeless misery envelopes me like a cold blanket of sorrow.

Oh how I wish it would set my spirit free and help me make it through until tomorrow.

I do not believe in God even though I think I should.

When they plant me beneath the sod will my soul and my spirit be there for good?

If I should succumb to this despair and forfeit the chance to reach my goal,

If it was too much for me to bear please take mercy on this coward's soul.

Don't ask me why but I feel a bit better after writing that; weird aye? It's much easier to pour it out on the page than to a human heart. I guess in a way I am pouring it out to you when you read it. Make of it what you will.

Tomorrow will be another day like yesterday and today; me sitting and staring down the lake and wondering. I certainly do not like being in limbo. I tell myself not to think too far ahead because it only gnaws at me more and more. I wonder if the doctors think about their patients and what they are going through or are they too busy with too many patients. I wonder if it would be rude to ask the doctor next week . . . if they don't cancel my appointment. Wouldn't that be a real test of one's metal? Then what would I do? OH I know, sit and fret until the next call. I still have six days until I see the doctor so I better not get ahead of myself.

Today is June the forth. It was forty years ago today I hired on with the railroad. Where has my life gone? Today will be for reminiscing I think. And it is perfect day weather wise to sit beside the lake and reflect back. It shouldn't be too difficult to use mind control today.

WOW! I just thought about something else; eighteen days until our forty third anniversary. I know Carol will forget it again this year just like she does every year. She is not any good at remembering dates. I'm not blaming her I'm just stating a fact. I'd like to take her somewhere special to celebrate but of course who knows where I'll be on June the twenty second. Well this year I'm not going to let the threat of cancer stop us from having a good time on our anniversary; so much for mind control.

My first reminiscence about our worst time together brings tears to my eyes because it has been a long time since I've thought about losing our son Jason when he was only eight months old. Up until he passed away I had never even heard the word, "Meningitis." I guess I have to get the sad thoughts over with before I can move on to the good ones. Maybe it's time for me to give thanks for the length of time I've had the pleasure to be alive. I have to stop writing for a while as it is too hard on me when I keep coming back to talk about death.

Usually for me it does no good to look back. Looking forward makes it easier to have positive thoughts. Both our children and their children are all health and doing well. And of course we have the great grandchild on the way. What a shmuck I am to sit here and fret over my setbacks when there is so much happiness all around me. I should be ashamed of myself.

My brother in law Gary just arrived in camp. The first words out of his mouth spoke of death. Apparently his cousin was killed in Auckland in an explosion; so much for thinking happy thoughts today.

I've been thinking about the possibility of smoking pot again. It's been a few years since I was told to give it up. I didn't want to but someone thought it best I do and she knows best. I found it helped me look at life from a less serious view. Of course if I did start smoking pot again it would not help the seriousness of the friction it would cause between Carol and me. I guess I'd best scrub that thought and move on to the next one.

Okay . . . For a day where I was supposed to be happy I'd say things are turning out fairly normal. I've come to the conclusion you cannot escape reality. A famous poet once said, "No man can escape by hiding behind the door of reality, for reality will be the first thing to greet him when he comes out."

Rob and Melisa just walked down the road from their campsite with Rob's grandson. Rob is a recovering drug addict. Having his grandson with him he said, "Today is a good day . . . Tomorrow, now that's another day." He still thinks one day at a time and today is his good day.

I did not want to get out of bed this morning. All I wanted to do was stay curled up in a ball next to Carol. Sometimes the safest place for the mind to be is tucked away under the covers. But . . . I did get up and went through my routine once again. There wasn't a cloud in the sky and it looked like it was going to be a great day. I'll just have to wait and see how things develop. At the very least it looks like it's going to be a nice quiet Sunday.

Sometimes when I sit in my lawn chair I take a pen and paper with me to write down a poem that forms in my mind. This morning I watched a rather large bald headed eagle gliding over the water in search of its breakfast.

Oh bold bird of bliss and sombre pleasure, grand master of airy space.

Where all below is unclaimed treasure; and me, a sky my eyes to trace?

On distant hills his shadow falls, a path of greying subtle light.

Swiftly, swiftly, all nature calls; and me, steadfast in my plight.

Upon the wind he mysteriously steals, in silence a beating heart to pound.

Oh splendid creature how it feels; and me restored to humble ground.

Such freedom is his daily feast, and his flight the jealousy of my eyes.

On the wind he is a scentless beast; and me alone beneath spacious skies.

Through weeping clouds and sunset hour, and in the mist of waking morn;

Oh bold bird of altitude and awesome power; and me melancholy and forlorn.

His wings impatient like the breeze, this wanderer of cloudless climes.

And all he feels and all he sees; and me on the landscape of sadder times.

High heaven holds his cloudy breath and languishes in his secret heart.

A silent sky could not endure your death; and me this earth cannot depart.

I envy him his freedom as he lifts a silver fish from the water and returns to his nest across the lake. I'm sure his family is anxious to see him. I smile to myself and pull my cap down over my eyes to have a nap and perhaps dream of such freedom.

I never managed to nap this morning. I was too busy listening to Carol and Dawn talking about cheese. I think they named every cheese known to man. One thing led to another and they started talking about the past. Of course that made me start thinking back. My mind for some unexplainable reason went back to when I was twenty two, before I met Carol. I haven't told anyone this in many years but I spent three weeks in an institution outside of Vancouver. Some refer to it as a place for troubled souls. Apparently I didn't know the difference between sex and love. The one thing I remember vividly is the Psychiatrist that I talked to. After listening to him for a short period of time I thought maybe he was one of the patients. All he told me was there are more than one fish in the sea. Now how profound is that?

It now seems ironic that in my youth I tried to kill myself and now in my senior years I'm worried about death. What the hell is wrong with me, I should just make up my mind. I still have the visible scars on my wrists from those days but thankfully there are no emotional ones. It took me a while to sort things out but in the end I managed.

Now, where was I? Oh yeah, me and my positive thoughts. I haven't told Carol that I love her in a long time, nor has she told me. Are our lives so mundane that we forget what makes each other special? I know my frustration and anger stop me from doing and saying certain things once in a while. It's like I'm guarding myself against some unknown enemy.

Ten

Yesterday was priceless; we golfed with Gary and both Carol and I had great games. We had a wonderful lunch on the patio at the clubhouse and then came back to camp to sit in the shade and look down the lake. We had a couple of drinks before I started the campfire. It was such a great day I decided not to write about it yesterday because later when I did think of the "C" word I refused to let it wreck my day.

Today Carol is in town golfing ladies day. Today I am constructing a measuring device to let us know how much the lake goes up and down. I'm thinking of putting directional signs on my measuring post and perhaps a weather vane. Not only will it let us know about the water level it will let boaters know where north and south are. This is going to be fun. I'll let you know how it turns out when I'm done.

My measuring post will measure in feet because I'm too old to be a metric guy. I hate metric measurements; always have. As the water is down right now I'll take it just beyond the edge and weight the base down will large heavy rocks to keep it from tipping over in rough weather.

It took me the better part of the morning to finish it and it looks damn fine sticking up out of the water. I have one question though; why would a man of my age be so proud of something as stupid and simple as that? All it is, is a painted two by two with foot increments on it. Near the top is a sign that reads, "NORTH", and points in that direction. At the very top is a solar light. We wouldn't want any boats to smash into it a night now would we? Now what will I do with my waiting time? I'll think of something, I always do.

Tomorrow we have to get up at six in the morning because we have to be at the doctor's office in Salmon Arm by quarter to nine. I'm never late . . . ever.

I have it in the back of my mind he's going to examine the lump in my neck and tell me to come back next spring when it's a bit bigger. In a weird sort of way that would be fine with me. At least I could get on with my summer. I guess we'll find out tomorrow.

The sun never paid me a visit once today. But it was a nice quiet day and I had plenty of time to snooze and write poetry. I have to go to town in an hour and give golfer Carol a ride back to camp.

I slept surprisingly well last night. Carol was up very early because she said there were mice in the ceiling. When I said, "I doubt it" she became angry at me. I should have kept my mouth shut I guess. We're off to see the doctor in ten more minutes.

. . . . . We just got back from the doctor and I should be elated with what he said. However I think all we have done is postpone my apprehension. He said he should do a biopsy but wasn't too sure he could get a good sample because the lump is rather small yet. I suggested we wait and he said, "You must have read my mind. Let's take the advice of the CT scan people and do another CT scan in three months."

It was his opinion after feeling around my neck that it probably isn't cancerous. At first I was extremely happy to hear those words then I remembered that's what he said last time. At least now I can get on with my summer and lose some of the stress that's been plaguing me lately. I think Carol will like that also. I also realize it may affect my winter plans depending on what happens three months from now. Until then I am going to do my best to forget about it and enjoy Carol's company and a long hot summer.

Glen and Nelly arrive today with their (Big Ass Bus) motor home. I always enjoy their company around the campfire. Glen was happy because he managed to catch a few fish from shore in the four days they were here.

I realize how important it is to have friends that one can enjoy and learn from. Like the couple we met on the golf course in Yuma last fall. We became good friend over the winter and Carol and I always looked forward to Eva and Doug's company. Some people you meet just make you feel comfortable and this couple is one of those. When we parted ways in April I gave Eva a few of my stories to read, thinking she might like them. Lo and behold unbeknownst to me she was a documents editor in her working life. She has since then been editing my stories and I am so grateful for that. She probably thought I somehow knew she was an editor when I gave her my stories but I had no idea at the time. I think it was just meant to be. I know my stories read much better after she's had a go at them. Now if we could just find a way to make some money off of them.

Update:

It's been ten days since I've seen my doctor and I can truly say I'm stress free for the mean time. I did get a very bad case of gout for the first time in my life and let me tell you it is very painful. I think it was from all that stress but there are those who think it is because of my drinking.

I have had a couple of great compliments on some of the stories I've had published from two of the campers that read them. Even though Carol was sitting right beside me when they said how good they were she still refuses to read even one. I say I don't care but inside I do care. Of course by now even if she were to decide to read one I think it is too late to care what she thinks. She would only be doing it out of the curiosity of wondering why some like my writing. I'm over that now. The weather is still terrible and summer is almost upon us.

Oh! By the way, I did buy Carol that single red rose. She admired it for a few seconds and then said thanks and gave me a kiss. She never looked at the card where I had written, "I love you." Of course that's what the meaning of the single red rose is, but still it would have been nice if she'd have read the card. I got the feeling that it gave me more pleasure to give her the rose than it did her in the receiving of it. I suppose I'm over reacting. Maybe she thought it was long overdue and I can't blame her if she did.

The nerve of some animals; a young moose just walked out of the bush onto our shore line and it made Carol's day. Now, if a caribou would do the same thing then she would be extremely happy. She's never seen a caribou in the wild.

Eleven

Here it is almost the longest day of the year and we have yet to have a good stretch of sunshine. Maybe July and August will bring us what we want.

Today is June the 21st, one day before our 43rd anniversary. Also it's ladies day at the golf course. I get the day by myself in camp. Oh how I love these days.
I anchor myself to the shore with thoughts of sunshine on my mind.
I let my wandering mind soar and leave my troubles far behind.
I am a contented solitary soul enjoying this quiet time and place.
Today it is my individual role to keep a smile upon my face.

Today I am plagued by a bad back. It hurts just to bend over. I swear I must be getting old. My gout seems to have gone away, for now at least. I try not to do too much so my back can heal but there is stuff I must do. I don't want to pack this lifestyle in just yet.

June the twenty seventh and we golfed nine holes this morning. My back is a bit better but I had to quit after nine.

Today carol is golfing ladies day. I am a poet once again. My individuality restored to what it should be. I live today a happy camper free of pain, my heart is worriless and free. My neighbours are my kind of campers; we all get along amazingly well. Oh sure the odd time I need my dampers, just to stop from telling some of them to go to hell.

I sit in front of the trees along the shore and give names to each and every one. I sit here at nature's wide open door devising a tale and how it should be spun.

My kingdom surrounds me like a blanket for the soul;
As I listen to the ripples against the shore.
Nature in all her splendour fresh and whole,
My heart could ask for nothing more.

Strange how a man can just sit and think so clearly when he puts his mind to it. I love the freedom of this place and the peacefulness it provides. Tomorrow will come and take me out of myself and I will be just a little more tolerant of things.

Today has taken me back to this reality that I now must accept. My mind is addled with thoughts of death today. Don't ask me why because I have no idea how these things work. I think it was the news on TV that got me to thinking again. Of course those low dark clouds only aid in thoughts of gloom and sadness as they hang over our camp threatening to dump a ton of moisture on us.

Carol is working on her millionth crossword puzzle, all snuggled up on the couch in her house coat. Me . . . I'm uncomfortable with my thoughts today. I hope I get out of this funk that I'm in; I guess only time will tell. I keep my secret fears locked away in my heart. My moods seem to swing with the weather. I need some sunshine in my life. Depression is not a fun thing.

It's been a few days since I last wrote. Today is July the first and the weather is still not cooperating. I need some sunshine in my life. Dawn and Gary are in camp for a few days so that should help my mood.

Today is July forth and my son and his wife came out tonight to fish for a couple of hours. When they were done Shelly handed me a piece of paper. When I opened it and read it I found out I go back to Salmon Arm on August the third for another CT scan. I hope I'm not going to dwell on it too often. I will do my best to put it to the back of my mind for as long as I can. We had a great night around the campfire.

Today Carol's in town golfing with some other ladies. Today I decided to smoke marijuana for the first time in a long, long time. The only reason I have it is another story.

This person, who shall remain nameless, claims he found it on the golf course. Apparently none of the other golfers would own up to just whose it was. SOOO . . . this nameless person gave it to me. He told his story about it around the campfire and got quite a chuckle from the other campers. Of course I told them I was going to smoke it . . . Totally! Of course there was another titter or two. As it was mostly just the remaining dust left in the bag I doubted that it would be any good. Well I so totally have to tell you it is damn good. Nothing makes me want to write a poem more than being stoned. I hear the trucks and cars above me on the highway. I think I'll write about that.

They drive up and down the road, the workers; they do it daily for pay.
I'm what you call one of those shirkers, me, I just sit and wile away the day.
They have their hammers and their axes, they toil even when they're sick.
No one ever relaxes, except me . . . I'm kind of a lazy old prick.
They rise early and quit late, hard work is their common link.
Some would say that's just great, not me, I'm somewhat of a sluggish dink.
They have their hopes and dreams, as most workers would.
Not is always as it seems, take me; I'm no God damn good.
They drive up and down the road, the almighty dollar their goal.
They carry a pretty heavy load, not me, I'm a slothful soul.

WOW! Rather good if you do ask me. Yeah it's good stuff. But enough is enough. I never did smoke that crap . . . I was just having you on. I knew it would be no damn good so I threw it in the fire two nights ago and no one even smelt it burning. Now that's gotta tell you something you'd think. No, I just love to be left alone when I write poetry. I can`t have any negativity around me at all. When the time is right it`s like I`m under a spell; my mind goes to another place.

I found the worry stone my granddaughter gave me last year; I'm a changed human being. I remember how well it worked after she gave it to me. I seemed to me if an eleven year old girl thought I needed a worry stone; then hey, who was I to argue with that. Oh sure, as you all know, I still worry quite a lot but at least I don`t worry about the petty things anymore. Thanks Madi.

Twelve

My writing is getting better every time I write thanks to Eva. Thanks Eva, I can't repay you for your kindness except to simply say thank you. I know hardly any of my books sell because they get no exposure; I've known since the beginning.

You know . . . . Some of the humming birds around here are getting too fat and lazy. They guard the feeder and won't let any other humming birds feed. I think I've devised a plan to change that. I've decided I'm going to put out another feeder; that'll teach him a lesson.

Things gather in my mind and I write them down. I never know what it will be.

A humming bird just flew through my syllables; tickled my ear when it went by. I fish my words from a pool of syllables and fat adjectives. I look up and see wild horses with cloudy manes making their way across my sky. Out here I feel inconsequential. I am only an incident. Afternoon, get a grip on yourself; stop doing this to me. I watch as one who is evaporating into tomorrow; I am an absorbed human being.

Oh! It's time to go inside and make my lunch.

Lunch was a toasted bagel with cold beans and wieners; quite good actually. Now, where were we . . . Oh yeah, how easy it is to get lost in this place.
I name myself, tomorrow; I am a mile wide and mountain thick. At mid day a flock of birds freckled my sky; them and their mass of hasty appointments. This landscape surrounds me; I wear it like a tunic of green and blue. Nature is a gracious host; I hold her in high esteem. I feel if I close my eyes I will disappear. Here I will never grow old; I'm too tangled in her roots. I cherish this day. I just now discovered black flies cannot be discouraged by waving my words at them.

It's time for me to take my Fuji and go do some photography of flowers. The sun is bringing out all their great shapes and colors. I'll be back in an hour or so.

You might as well leave too!! Away you go . . . I'll let you know when I'm back.

There is a certain speciality that I feel when I see the sun peak over the mountain every morning. I also feel it is my duty to convey the importance of a great day. I did go up the road and photograph those flowers like I said I would. The Indian paint brushes are magnificent and bold with their dark red colors; and the daisies, man, there's millions of them.

It will be hard to leave this place. I'll have to make up a poem about it. I'll call it embarking.

If you think I am embarking, I am not embarking; I am merely pretending I have departed.
Even the wind pulls me along, pulls me out of this resplendent space through the window of my dreaming.
The night sky burps forth glimmering stars where patches of light explode with remarkable brilliance.
I go out when the moon is new and carry the stars on my shoulders.
I am an embarking stranger in these new fields of golden light that flourish above my darkness.

I am afraid to relax as I look down; I cannot conquer this fear that I have avoided for too long.

The ground is covered in a patchwork of silent surprises.

A newborn night is harmless and cheerful for a while; Then it begins to demand all the limits of me.

I fear my shadow will be stolen; I simply cannot give up my shadow to the turning moon.

I am a sequence of thoughts leading away from here.

I never expected to be a captive voyager pirouetting through space; yet!

I am this silent audience expected to applaud this procession of time.

I am here, I am breathing, and I am.

I have reached out with my imagination to dust off the stars of heaven.

If you think I am embarking . . . I am not embarking, I am merely envisioning departing.

As for today I have smooth sailing. It looks like sunny days ahead. Smooth sailing and a sky full of sunshine from now on. Summertime has graced this place with its splendour. Welcome summer, come on it and make yourself comfortable. Stay as long as you like, feel free to just be yourself. Take your time before you have to disturb my happiness. Make it so I'll miss you when it's time for you to depart.

I've come to the conclusion this place is changing me. We are alike; we both have our seasons.
I am who this summer is making; this shy monster beginning to understand that in life one must release the roar.
I must surrender to this nameless moment; this consequence of destiny waiting for the impatient clouds of summer to turn the seasons.
No tomorrow no yesterday, just this naked awakening.
I have dressed myself with this veil of my obligation.
I have drawn it about me like the calmer clouds of July and it is everywhere inside of me.
I am this silent joy, like summer clouds crumbling to the vague voice of autumn sun.
I am poet, poem, poetry, drifting freely like the lonely clouds of autumn not yet possessed by that harsher reality.
I am who this fading summer has made and all it has done is most meaningful.

Today we have our youngest granddaughter Madi visiting us for a couple of days. We just returned from a short canoe ride up the lake. We had a great day and a nice campfire. Of course Madi's not my little girl any more, she's becoming a beautiful young woman.

Well I guess we've had our two days of nice weather because it rained all night last night and the wind is blowing up the lake this morning. As I look out the window I can see my neighbour's boat knocked my weather station over.

As he has it on a bungee like cord and anchored on the bottom of the lake, the wind pushed it into my weather station and destroyed it. I knew it was going to happen.

This afternoon I decided to feel that lump in my neck. It definitely has grown as I no longer have to search to find it; it's easy to find now. Oh well, August the third and I'll have a better idea. It looks like we'll be spending another day inside. I was hoping to sit outside in the sunshine.

Since we've been given notice we may have to move from our campsite we all keep waiting for the forestry guys to come and lay the law down. Apparently some disgruntled campers from Revelstoke have complained we are having way too much fun. And then there's the gossip from those busy bodies with nothing better to do than sit around and drink coffee and expound on things they know nothing about. Most people that complain don't even camp. I guess we'll just have to wait and see what insane policy the forestry will come up with.

It's been raining and blowing for five hours steady. I fear I am suffering from ennui. See how bored I was; I went and found a word to describe how I felt. Now that is boredom at its finest if you ask me.

Thirteen

The more I think of it, I've come to the conclusion I should just build my life on today; what will be will be and probably tomorrow still will come. As for today I live in the freedom of the sun and the warmth of my wife. I have my happy hours, and certainly do have my sad. I think I fret on one thing too long and it takes all my focus. I try not to but I think that is the battle I shall not win. Who'd a thought that the mighty Peter would sweat such a little thing? I'm glad they really don't know me, because I am just like you and all the rest. Oh well! At least I'm still talking about it; that must mean something. I hope some of you don't think of me as a coward . . . because I'm not. Of course it's something you can't understand until you experience it; that's just how it is. I don't ask for your pity but I would like some understanding.

God knows I try not to cry when others are around, even though many times I wanted to. I held my tears back, it's not like I'm not trying. It probably is my own fault for putting everyone on, all my life; convincing them I'm strong and funny when in actual truth I'm not. I only tell you this now because sometimes I really do need someone to talk to. You don't mind do you?

 I think, just by writing my thoughts down I see it as my therapy. I feel like I can express myself fully when I'm not face to face. I just hope my wife reads this because she understands about my writing down my feelings; like the feelings I have for her. She knows she's my anchor; she's the star that guides my ship. She knows I couldn't survive without her. I can't tell you how many times she's turned my tears into a dazzling liquid river. Her love gives new meaning to the timeless dreams of love. She knows how much I love her.

 There are a few who will miss me when I'm gone. At least I hope there are some. Of course there are those of you who will say something like; "Well! At least he was on the other side of sixty five. He had a fairly good life." What if I was forty one, would I have lived a good life? The part of my mind that deals with this does not know about time. Age has nothing to do with it; we all want to live as long as we can.

I have to go pick Carol up from town, so thanks for listening to me. I do feel a lot better now. I think I'll tell her my writing went rather well today. There; therapy session is over.

This morning when we woke up we could hear some birds chirping outside our window. Their early morning lilting was a great introduction to the day. When Carol opened the blind to look out the sun poked her in the eye. I think canoeing is in our immediate future.

. . . . I woke up this morning having slept rather well. I give thanks to my writing from yesterday; today I carry a more positive attitude with me. We sat on "The patio" as we call it, and had our coffee as the sun was rising. We will go canoeing today.

Fourteen

It's been a few days since I've written anything. I think
that's good, don't you. We golfed yesterday and had a
great time. Carol chipped in from the rough on seven.
We had a great time. Today is the day we brave taking
the canoe across to the other side of the lake. We don't
want to get caught in a storm on the other side.
Sometimes we take a chance and it works out just fine; I
think today is going to be one of those days.

. . . .We just got back from the other side of the lake
and the water stayed dead calm for us both ways. We
had wondered where the beavers had gone that were

here last year, because they're not here. We think we discovered there new lodge on the other side of the lake, just south of the creek. We can't be sure but we think it might be them. Of course they told us to go away so we left them alone. We also spotted the bald eagle and found out where his new nest was. This year he made it bigger and built it higher. It was one of those perfect days that will be long remembered . . . by both of us.

Time is getting closer for me to my date with that scanning devise. It doesn't bother me very much anymore. We'll take things as they come from now on. I know you can't change what will be, so I just let it be. Our great grand daughter is going to make her grand entrance into our world. Now there's something to look forward to.

Today I'm going to tell you a secret I have never told anyone before. If I asked you to keep it a secret could you? Would you? You have to understand I find it difficult to open up to strangers but I'm starting to think of you as more than that. I feel I almost know you, because you obviously care, or you wouldn't still be reading this.

My secret has to do with when I was a child. My parents told me if I wondered too far into the woods around our farm alone the bad man would catch me. Even today I still have trouble walking alone in the woods. Don't parents know that little children believe in the boogieman? I don't like people thinking I'm afraid of anything.

You know when I started writing this story I had no idea where it would take me. I feel like I'm a general leading an army of words to wipe out my fears. I fear I will lose you and what you offer me; you who know me pretty well by now. I sense you might want some drama in my life so your reading will be much more thrilling; maybe when we get to the part where they tell me my cancer is back; that might make more interesting reading. We'll just have to wait and see.

Fifteen

I have some serious concerns about our life style and how it might have to come to an end. I think Carol is with me when I tell you we don't want to give up living in our fifth wheel. This is our home and we love it. But the forestry might just come along and tell us to move on. I hope not; at least not until next year. I love it here.

. . . . . It's been six and a half days since I last put words upon this page; nothing new to report; good days and bad days. Some people caught too many Kokanee and some never caught enough. Me, I caught two for Carol (because she loves them) and she gave them to her sister Dawn. She told me that dawn was pretty disappointed with Gary for not catching fish like all the others. It became quite the joke around camp for a few days.

We have some new campers beside us. They are locals and we know them; they're probably our kind of people. At least they seemed that way around the campfire last night. Once again it is Tuesday and Carol is golfing and me, I'm writing.

I'm trying to quit drinking again. This is the nine millionth time. I have to keep trying because if I don't then I'll have given up. I once went three weeks without a drop of alcohol. I think there's still hope. It's pouring buckets outside right now. It does sound good on the slide out.

Hi, it's me again. I know I've been ignoring you and you're probably angry with me for not getting to you sooner. I know it's been four days since I last wrote; and a long four days it was.

Great news arrived via Facebook that our great granddaughter Karlie Irene Rae has entered our lives. She weighed a healthy 7 pounds and 3 ounces. Everything went well and mother and child are feeling great. Me, I feel so old now that I'm a great grandfather. Where did my life go?

My older sister Ruth came for two and a half days. She's from Calgary and I love her dearly, but I was happy to see her go. We had a great visit. It's not that I don't like her company it's just our fifth wheel is too small for three people any more. Carol and I need our space now, so from now on no more company.

My sister falls asleep all the time. When you go to talk to her you have to look at her first to see if she's still cognisant. She's always been like that but now I think it is getting worse. She slept for three hours after super on the couch; sitting up. Then she went to bed and slept all night. What's with that?

I was late getting back today because her two o'clock ride never showed up until four thirty seven. I was a bit perturbed. Of course she forgot to get their cell phone number so she could phone them; no, that would be too simple.

Tomorrow I go for my CT scan. I'm not the least worried about it anymore but I will if it becomes a concern. Everything is picking up at camp what with the sunshine we've had lately. Everyone is getting along splendidly; we're all one big happy family. Today I sat out in the sunshine and listened to some music. It filled my heart with gladness. I couldn't help but write this poem.

Today I flew high on the wing with some of God's creatures.
I soared with the eagle and looked through his eyes.
They allowed me the pleasure to see all their finest features.
But all too soon it was time to say my sad goodbyes.

I sit in the lap of night wondering and waiting for tomorrow.
I shall rush headlong into it with the same gusto I did today.
I anticipate what it has to offer, be it happiness or sorrow.
But of course I'll have all the sweet memories of yesterday.
Goodnight; see you tomorrow.

I had my CT scan a few days ago; I probably won't know anything for a couple of weeks by the sounds of it.

I hope its sooner! It's not that I'm all that worried; it's just that I'd like to get it behind me. We're going to Sicamous tomorrow to visit our great granddaughter Karlie Irene Rae. I'm really looking forward to it.

Today the sun is peaking out over the lake and it looks like it may be a beautiful day. We have some new people in camp today . . . well, old new people. Glen and Barb are back to quench their appetites for fresh Kokanee. They'll share a place around our fire and we'll all sit and chat.

Glen and Nelly are back for a couple of days and it's nice to see they're both doing fine. Tonight's fire might be something to look forward to.

Guess what? It's Tuesday again and I am in camp alone to write. Today I will write on this page as though it were my plain of indifference.

Finding words for my poems is easy. I just sit beside the lake and they come to me like hummingbirds to their feeders.

Yesterday I thought about a lot of things. Today, for some unfathomable reason I find myself thinking about the hereafter. Don't ask me why because I don't know. I suppose if I were to make my peace with ... God, I'd have to tell him I believe in him. But if I believed him wouldn't he like me and make my cancer go away.

Dear Lord please forgive me for being such a sinner;
I now see too late in my life the glory of the truth.
Dear Lord I am so ashamed and honestly sorry
that I never gave you a chance back in my youth.
Dear Lord why didn't you show yourself sooner?
It would have saved us both a lot of grief.
Dear Lord thank you for showing me the light,
and most of all thank you for restoring my belief.
Dear Lord I guess that's all for today,
but as you can see I'm changing my thinking.
Dear Lord I'm starting to see the light;
my disbelief in you is definitely shrinking.

Dear Lord, forgive me ... just in case!

This afternoon I sat in my lawn chair and stared down the lake; sky, wind and water . . . and me. This is my paradise.

Sixteen

It's not all that busy this weekend at our spot. I think many campers have given up; too bad because the weather is at its finest. Tomorrow Carol and I are going canoeing. We're much more comfortable in the canoe this year.

.... It has been almost two weeks since I had my last CT scan and no one has contacted me about the results. Maybe having cancer is not that big a deal to the doctors anymore. One would think that they would get a hold of me and say something ... anything that may ease my mind would be nice to hear. Maybe I'll just tell them all to go to hell and not do anything until the lump gets so big I can't stand it. When it was big the last time it really got their attention.

When I went outside this morning I could feel the autumn chill in the air, and here it is only the middle of August.

Today I am writing a poem about a poem:

These black fragments of my grief rest in sentences that never end.
Words twisting, twisting out of my pen; the rhythm of my life cannot master them.
I have dreamed extraordinary poems; only to pour them out into a mere handful of expressions.
I am a freedom come to lead you on.
I am a tree stripped of the fruit of imagination; I am now nothing but paper.
There is more to a poem than what is left after it has been dismembered by your eyes.
This poem knows that you are necessary and it is less solitary.
It is your busy eyes that give it life.

What should it do if you were not here? But for you it alone must bear the burden of accomplishment. This poem does not yet know of death yet it will come through your eyes when you take your leaving.
It waits for so meaningful a rare visit.
Rise up and go. This poem has just ended . . .

There, now I feel better. It's time to go make myself some lunch.

Seventeen

Every once in a while I feel I have to tell you
something about me that I really do not want to tell you. I
suffer from depression every now and then; I have for
many years. On some occasions Carol confuses it with
pouting and on some occasions she's right.

I have been depressed for almost a week now and no
matter what I think or do nothing changes how I feel. I
wish I could just climb into a big box and close the lid and
stay there forever. I will sit in my lawn chair and stare
down the lake and if any one comes to talk to me I'll be as
pleasant as I can.

The way I'm feeling has nothing to do with cancer; although when I think about the possibility of my cancer returning while I'm depressed, I really don't care one way or the other. I have a complete lack of enthusiasm for anything. I am a body and mind deprived of will. Tomorrow we are supposed to go golfing. The last time I golfed when I was depressed was like sleep walking; you're there but you're not there. I know I can't just sit in camp all day every day and watch the month go by. I'll wait and see what tomorrow brings. I have thought about suicide in the last five days, on more than one occasion but I know that is not the answer. The last thing I would want to do is make my family suffer for my misfortunes.

This will be the last thing I ever write as I've given up on writing novels and short stories. I know that what I write is good, there is simply no way I can market them without spending money I don't have. I might as well waste my time in other areas from now on. I am grateful to Wordclay publishing for what they provided. On the other hand I am extremely disappointed with PublishAmerica for their lack of interest in helping me sell my novels. I guess this is just another one of those learning experiences that hopefully will make me wiser for the future. Time will tell.

I'm feeling much better today. I have no idea why because nothing has happened to change my mood. Perhaps it's just because that's how long my depression lasts and that is that.

We did golf the other day and I had my worst front nine of the year and then had my best back nine of the year; go figure.

Last night I had a most perplexing dream. I dreamt I was in a long line of slow moving people. I had no idea where the line was going and don't know if I knew any of the people. After a short time I could make out a long wooden box sitting on a stand about three feet of the ground. When I approached the one end of the box I looked inside and saw myself. I was dead and it never even startled me. As I walked away my mother took me by the hand and walked with me. She has been departed from this earth some two and a half years now.

I don't usually have dreams as vivid as that one. I'm sure it probably doesn't mean anything; well, I'm not completely sure.

It has been almost a week since I last put pen to paper and not much has changed. My golf game has not improved while Carol's has. I'm at the stage where I don't care about that lump in my neck. I have a half a notion to just forget about it until next year. It should have been addressed by now. My poem today is one that inspired me last night when I went outside to turn off the generator and looked up into a starry sky.
I call it

Extraterrestrial:

Crystal pin holes in the sky;
Night's sequenced gown.
A silken Moon drifting by;
night's enormous eye.
Threads of silver light flare;
Heaven's ennoble stir.
Each yet so perfectly rare;
Oh to be way up there.
A forever glowing wilderness;
the universes beating heart.
Nature's bold naked loveliness;
and my jubilation to confess.

A symphony of light and space;
a pilgrimage for the soul.
A mystery for Mortals to trace;
so many dreams to chase.
Secret secrets yet to measure;
so many nameless lights.
To sit and stare at this treasure;
a calm joy of instant pleasure.
Steep and lofty regions to climb;
seasonless to ephemeral man.
A paradise like frosted rime;
the unimaginable nudge of time.
Clusters in endless realms of sky;
a myriad of unexplainable forms.
A glimpse for Man's mortal eye;
And I can only wonder why.

Eighteen

Today is September the sixth. Tomorrow I go see my doctor in Salmon Arm about my last CT scan. I'm assuming he will want to do a biopsy; me, I'd rather just forget about it.

. . . . I just got back from my visit with the doctor. He gave me the news I wanted to hear. He is convinced that my cancer is NOT back and that is good enough for me. Today I am a forward looking man. Yesterday is forgotten.

Carol and I are looking forward to this winter in Yuma.

. . . . It's been almost five months since I last wrote. We are in Yuma and golfing with Doug and Eva. Life is great once again.

That lump has grown to twice the size of last September and once again I am concerned all over. I haven't said anything to Carol because there's no need for both of us to worry.

It will be the first thing I address when we get home . . . . Again!

I'll keep you all informed.

Bye for now.

PS I may have to write a sequel . . . . If that's okay with you?

Part Two

One

It's been almost a year and four months since I last came to write about my cancer. I suppose I should start by saying It's been a good year and four months. But now it is time to get back to addressing my problem. The lump in my neck is definitely getting bigger. Four days ago my doctor set up an emergency appointment with the specialist in Salmon Arm. Even then it won't happen for another twelve days.

Here we go again; waiting, waiting, waiting and fretting. It seems to me nothing ever changes. I worried yesterday and I worry today and certainly will tomorrow. My doctor thinks my cancer is back and I must agree with him. I wish there was some way to explain to you the anguish one goes through when faced with the uncertainty of the future. Words are not enough.

I never told anyone about my lump but I guess it was evident to a few people. To top it off I find out I have prostate concerns which are currently being addressed. I have to go to the hospital and have blood taken from me . . . again. I won't have any answer to that problem for a couple of weeks I would think. The stress sets one mind to thinking about all kinds of scenarios. All of them are not what one wants to think.

I was supposed to work at the golf course this summer but the club has no money to pay employees so that was another disappointment. Everything adds to my anxiety and it's hard to handle. I try not to get angry and control myself, especially with Carol. I wish I could just go somewhere and be by myself; I really do.

It seems to me the more I worry the more vivid my dreams are. Last night I dreamt I was walking down a gravel road which I had never been on before. When I came around a bent the road branched off in two directions. There was a sign post on the left hand one that said, "The end." The other sign said, "The end." I'm still trying to process what it really means.

This summer we have our fifth wheel in Dawn and Gary's yard. I know how lucky we are that they invited us to stay here. Of course staying up the lake is out of the question, what with the new rules and the fact our new fifth wheel is too big to get in and out of most of the camp spots. At least I know Carol will have someone to help her should I have to go for treatment. That is one worry less for me.

I read somewhere that when worrying becomes excessive it can lead to feelings of high anxiety and even causes you to be physically ill. I understand that all too well. I read another article that said excessive worrying affects your daily life so much that it interferes with your appetite, lifestyle habits, relationships, sleep, and job performance. Many people who worry excessively are so anxiety-ridden that they seek relief in harmful lifestyle habits such as overeating, cigarette smoking, or using alcohol and drugs.

I forgot to tell you after twenty some years of trying to quit drinking I finally did it. It's been fourteen months since I've had a drop of alcohol. I am most proud of that achievement. But lately I've been thinking what does it matter? Maybe drinking would help me relax and ease my fretting. Remembering back to the last time I think it didn't help me then and probably won't help me now.

I've pretty much given up on writing poetry. I think because now I'm in town and not up the lake I'm not inspired to think properly for the task of writing. Now I think of it I've quit doing a lot of things. Now my doctor tells me I should cut back on Caffeine, chocolate, acidic foods and a few other things because they are prostate irritants. I wonder where one should stop quitting things and just say to hell with it. I'm trying to stay positive and it works for a period of time but then my mood changes and I'm down in the dumps. I have thoughts that are not helping me to stay on a positive path.

On Monday morning I'm going to the hospital to have blood taken for my prostate problem. When my doctor phoned me to tell me to go and have that done he said, "No intercourse within seventy two hours of having my blood drawn." Then he said, "No ejaculating within seventy two hours." That really puzzled me.

I googled "Prostate blood test and ejaculation", and after reading the information was none the wiser. But then what do I know of such matters. Of course I'm anxiously waiting for Monday morning. I was going to go up to the hospital yesterday but I mistakenly took an allergy pill in the morning. Of course that screwed up the no eating or drinking for twelve hours prior to the blood sample. I am my own worst enemy. I wonder how long I'll have to wait for the results of the blood test.

Two

I play a lot of scrabble on the internet against other players. Many of them use a word generator program to make their words. I don't understand the reasoning for that. How can one get better at the game if they don't use their brain? Are they the ones who take the easy way at everything they do? If so, I pity them. When I accuse them of using a word generator most of them won't reply to that statement. I suppose there are a few out there who are extremely gifted and don't need a generator to win their games.

Today we are golfing and I hope it doesn't rain . . . again! Nothing takes your mind off of your worries like golfing. It demands your complete attention; much like fighting cancer does.

Yesterday was good; we enjoyed a rain free round of golf. Today the sky is bright blue. As I write this I still feel the anxiety of this waiting. I remember the last time all the feelings that engulfed me; helplessness, despair and a whole lot of depression. It's not all that easy to put it out of one's mind nor do I think that would be the answer even if one could. It is hard to make rational decisions when a person is overcome with muddled thoughts.

Today is June the seventeenth and I must go to the hospital for another blood test. Of course you know what that means! Time is slowly passing towards my date in Salmon Arm. I had a great father's day golfing with Carol and two friends. It's funny how I thought about cancer on the course every now and then but it didn't bring me down like it does when I'm just sitting around.

Last night I had trouble going to sleep. I started thinking back about Carol and I and how much I have disappointed her over the years. Once again I must say I know she deserves better than what I have given her; or should say what I haven't given her.

My dream last.

I went camping south of Revelstoke with some other people; who, I don't know. A short distance from our camp was a white-walled castle that towered very high above us. There were no doors or windows visible to me. Near the very top I could see it was old and crumbling. Beside the left hand corner high above me was the largest birch tree I'd ever seen. Somehow; as you can only do in dreams, I climbed up the outside to reach the top. When I stepped over the top I landed on a beautiful green lawn with beautiful people all over the place. One in particular was a young girl no more than ten years old wearing a white dress that puffed out over her knees. She was wearing something that held a small green tree over her head and when she walked it scraped the bottom of one of the arches. I remember thinking; who are they and what are they doing here? As I write this I now remember they cut down a large birch tree on the golf course!

Our forty fifth wedding anniversary is coming up in four days. Honest to God I do not know where the time went.

I miss waking up and looking down the lake. I can still picture it in my mind but that is not the same as being there. Often I wonder how Icarus and all the other humming birds are doing without us there. I named the dominant one 'Icarus" because he always flew the closest to the sun when he put on his displays. I hope they miss us as much as I miss them. I also wonder if the ospreys are back in their nest ready to raise a pair of young like they do every year; and the beaver that swam by our spot every night and returned the next morning. I guess we're all creatures of habit.

It saddens me to think of "The lonely guy." Every spring a large male goose would show up. We believed he lost his mate and will spend the rest of his life all by himself. I wonder what goes on in his mind. Is a half a life worth living? I think not!

One of the most fascinating displays we ever saw up the lake was when a bald eagle tried to take a fish away from an osprey. They swooped and rose out over the lake right in front of us. The eagle's persistence finally paid off when the osprey tired out and dropped the Kokanee and flew back to his nest. Of course the eagle flew down the lake to his waiting family. You just never know what will unfold before your eyes on that lake. It feels good to remember the good things in life. Someone once said, "Enjoy the here and now for all too soon it will only be a memory."

I started off the season by golfing for nothing because I was going to be an employee at the golf course. As time dragged on without getting hired, we came to an agreement that I would pay half the yearly dues and address the issue when I got hired on. It now looks like I will not be hired and have come to the decision I must quit golfing for the rest of the year. I think I should save my money just in case I have to fight cancer again. Of course if we want to go back to Yuma this winter then my health insurance premium will triple. We may not be able to afford to go. I hope Carol doesn't get too mad at me.

Today we went golfing . . . right after Carol criticized me; I hate golfing when I'm pissed off. I quit after nine holes. I see all the golfers out there using carts. Some need them and some think they need them. It's kind of an oxymoron; a healthy person golfing with a cart. Why even get off the cart, just drive up to it and reach out and tap it forward. And for some unknown reason the carts are driven right up to the edge of the green!

I think it's time to quit golfing until I get my health issues figured out.

Today is June twenty first, the day before our anniversary. I had planned to take Carol out for dinner tomorrow night but now I think it will not happen. I wish there was some way to get through to her that I cannot stand it when she criticizes me and talks down to me. I guess every now and then she has this need to piss me off.

Last night it rained the hardest I've ever heard. Today is our anniversary and I'm so pissed off from her criticizing me I doubt I will have much to say to her. I am so frustrated I do not know what to do. I do know one thing; it will never ever change. I must be such a disappointment to her; yesterday, today and tomorrow will be all the same.

Yesterday was our anniversary. The only words I spoke to her were, "I'm ordering pizza for supper." That was it. Today we golfed for the first time in three or four days. It was a good round. I wish Wednesday would hurry up and get here.

Last night I laid awake in the dark thinking about death. I came to the conclusion that when we sleep for hours that is a death of sorts. I think that is the way I'd like to leave this earth; fall asleep and never wake up.

My dream was a strange one. I was in a long, long line-up to get fed. When I got to the food there were no plates. I went in search of plates and came to an old door. It led to a basement where I found another door that took me down a dark corridor to a door that opened into a room with men sitting around. (Perhaps it was a waiting room . . . for you know what) I recognized one of the occupants and asked him if there was a way out other than where I came in; he pointed up. I climbed some old wooden steps and lift a floppy thin panel and saw nothing but large red ants. They were everywhere. I woke up before anything happened. From that dream I must conclude that I may have a few doors to go through and my way out is going to be in stages and not too pleasant near the end. The person I recognized was a guy I worked with on the railroad and to my knowledge is still alive.

Today I was quite proud of how I kept my composure on the golf course. Oh sure I swore after taking two doubles and was too mad at myself to swear when I took a seven on a par three. There was a time when I would give up and just finish the round, but not today. I ended up with nine pars to go with those doubles and that seven. In the end I shot eighty six. Maybe I'm getting the hang of dealing with adversity.

I never dreamt last night; at least nothing that stirred my memory; I slept rather well though. I was pretty disappointed with myself this morning and that's all I'm going to say about that. Of course it's raining out . . . again! Right now I'm operating on fifty percent of what my mood should be. Something has to happen soon to alter that.

My doctor just phoned and set up a "non emergency" appointment. I assume I don't have to worry about prostate cancer. That is good news. Maybe he can address my other problem with my prostate.

Last night I had a few dreams but the only one I vividly remember is Carol taking three tee shirts out of one of my drawers and told me which one to wear. Of course I could have been awake for that. I assume that dream was for what lay ahead later in the day. Today we go to Salmon Arm to see the specialist about that lump. Here goes!

Things went rather well at the doctor's in Salmon Arm. After he examined the lump in my neck he more or less agreed with me that the cancer is probably back. I go for a CT scan and a biopsy on July 16th. He also said I may have to go to Vancouver for a second opinion. I am of the opinion he will operate on me and extract the cancer. I cannot have radiation treatment again. I am surprisingly unworried now that I know more. I will now wait until the results of the biopsy are made. Of course that could be some length of time down the road.

Three

Last night when we went to bed I held Carol in my arms. My mind drifted off into a poem.

I feel the warmth of her sleeping breath; two hearts beating in perfect rhyme. Bother me not tonight death; I'm enjoying this moment in time.

I now find myself thinking about a few questions I should have asked the doctor yesterday. Like, if I can't have radiation again what will happen with my cancer once the lump is removed? Will it come back and have to be removed yet again? I'm sixty eight years old; will I be able to outlast its destruction?

No matter what, I've decided to focus on my health rather than the cancer. In order for me to maintain my health a positive attitude could be the difference maker. Writing helps my emotional health.

One of my biggest worries is will we be able to go to Arizona for the winter and if the answer is yes then will my insurance costs be too much? One thing at a time I guess!

It's hard for me to admit but I now know that anxiety has gripped me more than I thought in the last two weeks. My mood swings go from very down to medium down. Today I feel great and am ready to golf with Carol under blue skies. Tonight I plan on taking her out for supper.

We just got back from golf. I had one of my best games ever and am now a fifteen handicap on the Revelstoke course. I never would have thought in my wildest dreams to be that low. But now I feel comfortable at that handicap. Carol's a little disappointed with her game right now.

I've been reading about cancer and common questions asked by cancer patients. One question is, "Why me?" I've never asked that question; it seems almost silly to even think that. As my brother George would say, it is what it is." I have thought on more than one occasion how I'm glad it is me rather than anyone close to me.

Today is June 29th and when I woke up this morning I started thinking about the upside of me passing away. The first thing that came to mind was the fact I would not have to go through the grief of going through my sisters and brothers passing. Secondly, it may give Carol a chance to find someone who can afford her the chance to do the things she always wanted to do that we could not afford to do. That is my one regret in life; I never saved enough to fulfill Carol's expectations in retirement.

When I look at it one way I think I should be happy to have lived 85% of my expected life-time. That's more than most people in this world get. Our son Jason only lived for six months. My father lived thirty seven years, so why should I feel sorry for myself. Don't get me wrong, I know it will be extremely difficult near the end. After our son Todd was born I found myself going into his bedroom at night to make sure he was still breathing. Sometimes I would wake him up just to be sure.

I can't thank Dawn and Gary enough for providing us with a place to live and be worry free, which allowed us to live the life we wanted. Some people don't understand why we would want to live in our fifth wheel. We've never cared for large, expensive, grand surroundings. I would love to live the way we live until I die; oh wait, I am.

I don't like any negativity in my life; I never have; especially now what with the anxiety and the way my mind is going. Yesterday when they phoned from Salmon Arm to tell me the time for my CT scan, I had forgotten about the time for the biopsy on the same day. No big deal, right? Instead of Carol saying nothing, she said "I CAN'T BELIEVE YOU FORGOT THAT TIME." How negative and annoying is that. Later in the day while I was pouring ice tea some dripped on the counter top. She jumped toward the counter and said, "YOU'RE SPILLING IT ALL OVER THE PLACE; all over the place. . . Really? Of course she says it like I'm such a disappointment. I wish she could keep her negative thoughts to herself. Whenever she makes mistakes I never ever say anything negative. She on the other hand never misses an opportunity to let me know that I'm not perfect . . . I know that, so quit reminding me all the time.

I have one question nagging me and that is, what will happen after the surgeon removes that lump from my neck? The thought scares me.

I told my Daughter what was going on this morning. I wish I didn't have to tell anyone but I don't want my children to hear about it from someone else. It sounds so stupid to tell them not to worry. I haven't told my son just yet, although I did mention I had an appointment to see the specialist. At least the seed of possibility is planted.

Today is July the second and I told my son about my cancer being back. I handled it a lot better than the last time. It's hard to present a brave front when faced with such a terrible disease.

Today my word is, "Plotz." I am overwhelmed with emotion. I get that way when I'm all alone; too much time to think and worry. The more I dwell on it the more anxious I become. I can feel my mood changes and it scares me. It does not give one a good feeling not knowing what the future holds. Or should I say the immediate future. I don't know if what I'm saying will help anyone of you but I will tell you it's not helping me.

I'm no good at just sitting around; never have been. When I'm writing a novel it keeps my mind focused on the subject. But this writing is not like that . . . well I guess it might be! I feel so down this afternoon that I do not even want to talk to anyone. If you put a gun to my head I would not care. I hate this!

Given my depression yesterday I thought I would dream about death but I never. I tried to talk to Carol about my depression but when I started the words would not come out. I found myself getting ready to cry. It's a little early for tears, I would think!

I saw my doctor yesterday about my prostate problem. He says there is a chance of prostate cancer and I could have a biopsy on it. It sounded like it was painful and risky. We decided I would wait because of my other cancer problems. I will get it checked again in a few months; one problem at a time.

Last night's dream was stupid. I was golfing and used peanut butter for my tee. What the hell's with that? Today when I golf I will try not to dwell on my upcoming date in Salmon arm because it's still nine days off. I'm doing my best to stay positive. As long as I keep busy I'm fine.

Today is July seventh and I feel like such a wimp. Just what the world needs; another wimp! I think it's the rain outside that puts me in this funk of a mood. Waiting and waiting keeps me on the edge of my nerves. Also for the first time, that lump in my neck gave me a stinging pain.

While golfing this morning I told a friend about having cancer. I never know whether I should tell them or keep my mouth shut because I'm not looking for sympathy or anything like that. I guess once word gets out then everyone will know. This afternoon I sat in my lawn chair and felt sorry for myself. I sat in wounded silence staring upward as though some great sign would arrive out of the blue. Does a black raven count as a sign? I think it probably does. I hope I'm just being paranoid.

I fear it is almost time to quit golfing, at least until I settle what's going on in my life. I do not want to quit but I think I should save my money for what possibly lies ahead.

I never know when my disposition will change or what will cause it to change. My mood went down deep into the basement today; into the darkness that companions the soul. I do not know how long I must stay down in the depression of that hole.

Before I teed off on #14 today I thought to myself, "Why can't I just have a heart attack right now and get it over with." I know I'm not supposed to think like that but there's nothing I can do about my thoughts when I'm down. I don't have anyone who I can talk to about how I feel; at least no one who could understand my emotions.

Today is July the 16th and I just got back from my CT scan and biopsy. As I needed a fluid pumped through me for the CT scan the technician tried to stick the drip needle into my right arm three times before giving up and putting it into my left arm. She claimed there was too much scar tissue in the right arm from previous needles.

As for the biopsy, my doctor went to freeze the lump and it hurt terribly. When he stuck the bigger biopsy needle into the lump I almost passed out from the searing pain. Maybe there was no freezing fluid in the first needle. While I was trying to catch my breath he called me Tim. My name is not Tim, or Bill, or number thirty seven; my name is Peter and I'm important. After that I felt like I was just another person in a long line to be jabbed and sent on his way. Thanks doctor Killjoy.

The results will be back next week but he is almost certain my cancer is back. Even though he removed the last cancer he said this one is too complicated for him. He is sending me to Vancouver to see a neck and throat specialist. He said the specialist will set a time for me to go to Vancouver again for an operation. There they will remove the cancer, lymph nodes and some muscle tissue. The muscle tissue will be replaced from my chest muscle. There also may be complications with the blood vessels around the cancer. Of course the operation may not be until early September. When we exited the hospital I never made it to our truck before I started crying. I knew it was coming, I just didn't know how long I could hold it in. It is a helpless feeling to have no control over your life. I guess I'm back to a lot of anxiety and waiting again.

Four

I quit golfing yesterday because I had only paid half the dues. I'm not sure what expenses I will incur from here on. As much as I love golfing I must focus on a satisfactory end to my dilemma.

One would think at some point in time a person could accept what is going on in their life and get on with it; one would think! I am well aware of the fact that my being down also brings Carol down. How do I remedy that? Maybe I'm just a wimp and that is that.

I can't tell you about my dream this morning because it was sexual. But I will tell you it was delicious. I've gotten out of bed at four in the morning the last two days; too much on my mind.

Thank God Doug and Eva invited us to stay with them when I have to go to Vancouver, and for offering to get me to my appointments. That should reduce my anxiety by a bunch. I am so not a big city driver.

I now realize how mundane my life is without golf; more time to worry about things. Carol must be getting tired of my unhappiness but what can I do? I am the most depressed I've been in a long time and there seems to be no way to get out of it. I hate this feeling. I do not want to talk and I wish I were somewhere else. I do not know where that somewhere else would be.

I spent all of yesterday down in the dumps. Today is Saturday and Carol is golfing and going for lunch with the girls. Me, I would like to hike up into the bush and just sit there by myself. This sitting in limbo weighs heavy on my mind. I'm sure anxiety leads to depression. At least that's what has happened to me. I probably come across to Carol as being sad.

Maybe if I tell you something more about me that will make me feel better. Let me see . . . My mother ran a post office fourteen miles from the nearest town when I was in my early teens. We never had any money because she looked after five of us by herself.

A buddy and I built a dilapidated cabin in the trees about a quarter of a mile from our houses out of scrap wood and tin. We used old doors for the roof and it had one window. We never measured the window opening so we just took two windows from his farm that we thought would fit. Just before we got to the cabin I tripped and the window I was carrying broke. The one my pal was carrying fit rather well. We needed candles for light so we decided to steal some at the drug store in town. The first time I did it I was terribly afraid but soon found out it wasn't that hard to do. Once we realized we could steal that easily we moved up to stealing ammunition and cigarettes from the country store down the road from us. We would trade the ammunition for bottles of wine from the older boys. Two fourteen year old boys and two bottles of red wine made for a night of stupidity in our cabin. We never got caught but a friend did one time when he was with us and that scared the hell out of me. I never stole another thing from that day on. I'm not ashamed of what I did because that's the way it was back then.

We used to make money flipping for quarters at school. Once we found out that with a bit of practice we could distinguish the difference between a head or a tail just by feeling the coin with our thumbs it was easy. We would pretend we were playing each other at heads or tails and wait for someone to join us. Once someone said they'd like to play "Odd man wins" we would make sure I had a tail and he had a head. We'd switch every now and then. We did let the sucker win once in a while. Back then my nickname was Foxy. I guess that was because I was so sneaky and sly. But of course I had to be because of the bullies that picked on me. I was easy prey because I was the skinniest kid in school. You learn rather quickly to get on the right side of the wrong people.

Today is Sunday and I find myself alone as Carol is golfing. I sat in my lawn chair looking back on my life. It occurred to me that we all start out full of promise. But some of us for one reason or the other fall short of what could have been. I do not blame the fact that I was fatherless; god knows my mother did more than could be expected.

I started drinking at the age of fourteen and that continued until fifteen months ago when I somehow managed to quit cold turkey. But that was far too late. It seems that I spent my life just trying to get through life rather than thinking of the future and my duty to my wife and children. To say I am a failure is an understatement. I blame everything we do not have squarely on me.

Now what lies ahead financially I do not know; but I do know we will not be able to afford to go to Yuma this winter. That hurts almost as much as being told my cancer is back. Once again I've let Carol down. If we had any money to share I would like to ask her if she would like to leave me and get on with her life. Right now I could easily go somewhere to be by myself. Don't get me wrong; everything I've done and everything that has happened is totally on my shoulders . . . except cancer. I had no say in that.

Five

I guess it's time to tell you something more about me. When I was young I was bullied at school because I was the smallest skinniest kid in school. Later on when I was about twelve or thirteen I saw a big boy pushing a little boy to the ground. Something inside of me snapped and even though that bully was bigger than me I went to him and shoved him so hard he fell to the ground. I was scared and yet I yelled at him to leave that boy alone. He could see the anger in my face because he got up and walked away. I still to this day get a sick feeling in my gut when I think of it.

This morning when I woke up I had one thought; "I wish it was ten thirty at night so I could go to bed and circumvent the day". I don't look forward to sitting and staring at the blue sky. Maybe today I'll stare at the trees. I think I'm about two or three days from hearing from my doctor in Salmon Arm; I think? Of course I already know what he will say, but it will be time to proceed to the next stage of events. Time will once again slow down and anxiety will rise.

Today is one week since I saw the doctor. I'm expecting a phone call from him today or tomorrow. I will not hold my breath. It's like living in the shadows; the not knowing for sure. Oh well; time to go play some scrabble.

I've decided to start golfing again. It's too stressful sitting around and waiting. We golfed this morning and I was so glad to be out there. I never golfed very well but that didn't matter. This afternoon my doctor called and said the words I did not want to hear; "Your cancer is back."

Now I sit and wait to hear from the neck and throat guy in Vancouver. My doctor said if I don't hear from him in two weeks to call my local doctor. TWO WEEKS. . . When I told him I thought it would be soon he said, "Well, maybe he's on holidays." Oh! I'll just tell this growing lump in my neck to take a vacation. So, here I go again. . . Waiting!

I can fly. I did it again this morning in the dark behind my eyes. I often dream about me flying; not with wings, it's more like floating. I float above everyone and try to get their attention so they can see my great feat but no one ever looks up. I never associated my flying dreams with death before but this morning I floated so high all the people below looked like ants. Does that mean I'm getting closer to you know where? I'm not sure.

I've been waiting a week now to hear from the specialist in Vancouver. I wonder if they know that cancer is a serious thing. Perhaps I'm just one of too many waiting for assessment and treatment. Oh well! I'll just sit here and twiddle my thumbs. The lump is growing bigger. Now when I shave I have to go around it with my electric shaver.

This afternoon I sit in my lawn chair and stare at the sky. I am an Island in the middle of my marooned thoughts. Despair sits on the horizon behind me; my determination is for the future. Each day that passes strengthens my fortitude and toughens my spirit for the big fight. I am with one that must be. I close my eyes and compose myself into darkness. I think of what I must say for what lies ahead.

Now that I have departed life I thought you'd like to know; I still think of you dear wife, for your memory lives in my soul. I'll come to you in your sleep to ease the pain of your fears. Please do not worry or weep nor shed anymore tears. I now reside in the great beyond free from the calamities of life. My memories are sweet and fond all because you were my wife.

I phone the medical clinic for an appointment with my doctor. My doctor in Salmon Arm told me to get a hold of him if I don't hear from . . . . The phone just rang and I got my appointment in Coquitlam for the 7th of Aug. at 10:00am. Why am I choked up and have this lump in my throat?

Ye4sterday I decided to volunteer to work at the golf course because they are strapped for money. I'm not really the volunteering kind but thought I would try it. I told the superintendent i would show up at 06:00 AM today. When I arrived one of the staff said he would not be in today and they knew nothing about me being there. I guess it wasn't that important. If he needed volunteers you would think he'd let someone know about free labour! Never mind the fact that I got up at 05:00 AM. I'll be having words with him when we next meet.

All is forgiven; I went to work at the golf course today and drove a mower. It felt good to volunteer and do some good.

Last night I dreamt I was drinking a beer and after I drank it I realized that I had screwed up my no drinking policy. Image that; thinking that while dreaming it. It has been almost fifteen months since my last drink. When I woke up I was relieved to say the least.

Tomorrow morning we drive to Vancouver for my appointment with the doctor. We'll probably be on the road by six because it's the long weekend. I'll let you know how things go. Wish me luck!

Today is Aug. 06 and we are at Doug and Eva's in Langley. I am so thankful for their generosity and it makes me feel good to see Carol so relaxed here. Today we golf; tomorrow I see the specialist. I will admit I am nervous about what he will have to say.

Last night I dreamt that my Bro Jim and his wife Janice and my youngest Bro came to Revelstoke to wish me well! When I hugged Janice I wept. Bro John just walked by and went into the living room. It was in our old house in lower town. We haven't lived there for over a dozen years or more. Later today I will find out what is in store for me.

I just returned from the specialist's office. I will be going to Surrey Memorial Hospital for an operation to remove the cancer sometime within the next four weeks. Because I can't have radiation any more that will be it; how did he put it; "A one shot deal." I will be in the hospital overnight. There will be another visit to see him within two or three weeks of the surgery. There is still a chance we can go to Yuma for the winter.

Before we made it home the doctor's office called and said I will have surgery on Aug. 28th at Surrey

Memorial Hospital. That's good, at least now I know when and where. I will not be able to drive for at least two weeks after the operation so I'm hoping Gary will be kind enough to take me down and bring me back. I hate relying on friends and relatives but in this case I have no other choice.

If I dare say I would say that this doctor is going to rid me of cancer. It will be so great to have this over and just get on with my life. I know it's stressful on Carol as well. I'm not even worried about how long it will take me to get back to normal where I can golf again. Who knows, maybe I'll be able to keep my head down better after the surgery.

I think I'm on my way to recovery because everything is in place; date is set, place is set, ride down and back is set and most importantly I have a good feeling about it all. I'm ready and looking forward to the end of it all. If there's one thing I've learned since two thousand and six when this all began that is life means nothing without family and friends and the caring medical profession. I have met and had the support of everyone whom I met along the way. I definitely have a clearer view of what life should be all about. Thank you everyone.

Some days are just better than others; take today for instance. We went golfing with friends and Carol shot her lowest score ever. She shot eighty six. To me that is phenomenal. I matched my best game ever on the Revelstoke course; eighty two. After that my brother and sister from Alberta showed up and we went for a great lunch. No I ask you, does it get any better than that? I think not.

At this stage of events I have one thing to say about cancer. It can be just as emotionally devastating as physically. If you let it get to you then it will work against you physically; trust me I know. Everyone who is trying to help you will help you. But only you can fight the fight within your mind. Sitting around and fretting over it is the worst thing anyone can do.

Just before I woke up this morning I levitated. I was walking along a dirt path with yellowish grass along it and I rose up off the ground and went parallel. I was floating about four feet off the ground. I've done this before in dreams but this time I had trouble getting my feet back on the path. I had to use all my powers to stand firmly on the ground. Does this mean I'm getting ready to go somewhere?

We made up our minds yesterday; we are going to Yuma this winter. This morning I got another call on the golf course. I have a few pre-op meetings to attend at the Jim Pattison Surgical Center the day before my operation. I'm ready . . . bring it on.

I received an appointment with a specialist from Kelowna to have a video call at the Revelstoke Hospital on Tuesday the 25th; six more days of waiting. I'm beginning to wonder when the waiting stops and we get on with some answers and treatment. It's killing me inside.

Six

Today is August 20th and Carol is golfing ladies day. Me, I'm thinking about my surgery and looking forward to what lies beyond it. I just wish I didn't have to rely on family and friends to help me. But I guess I would do the same for them.

Yesterday I phone the specialist in Vancouver and found out my surgery time for the 28th. I must be at the hospital by 11:25 and the surgery will be about two hours after that. So that's it; everything is in place. It's time to buck up and move forward.

I'm starting to experience the grip of anxiety. I'm only three days from surgery and my worry level is on the rise. Of course I will not admit it to anyone but myself. If not for Doug and Eva's invitation to stay with them and be driven to the hospital by I think my apprehension would be unbearable by the time I arrived at the hospital. I am so grateful to Gary for taking time out of his life to transport Carol and I to Langley and back. These are the kind of acts one simply cannot repay; except maybe to recover and become a better person.

Today is August 27th and I'm finished with all the pre-op stuff. Tomorrow I go under the knife. The next day we will head back to Revelstoke.

This morning I woke up raring to go. Hospital here I come. I do find I am a bit antsy though. I found myself walking aimlessly around Doug and Eva's house a few minutes ago. And time; it do drag slowly when one is waiting for the important things. I won't be writing anymore until after I get back to Revelstoke.

We just got home from the operation. I was ready to tell you how euphoric I felt. But for some reason I feel like I'm still fighting. After we were home for a short time I held Carol and wept. I think that is because I was so focused on what I had to do that now it's over I just lost it. I'm having some discomfort and will be a while getting back to normal. But at least that lump is gone . . . again! Tomorrow is my day to try and forget.

I slept remarkably well last night; between my recliner and the bed. This morning I woke up feeling better. However after breakfast when I hugged Carol I had to hold back the tears. I'm having trouble understanding that but I suppose it's because she's the only one besides me that truly understands what I'm going through. It just makes me feel weak when I do that. I know I should be elated that it's probably over but every so often when I think about it I start to cry. Carol says it's normal and she's probably right. I suppose as the days go by I will look at life the way I should. I am grateful to everyone who helped me.

Each day I feel better, physically and emotionally. Today the sun is shining and I'm going for a walk later. I get a head ache after walking a block or two. I'll just keep at it and I'm sure the results will come.

It's day six after the operation and I feel myself healing. I don't sleep too long at any one time during the night. I start aching on my right side if I lay in one spot too long.

Yesterday my spirits were high; today, not so much. The right side of my head hurts, my right shoulder is aching but most of all my spirit has abandoned me. I fell like giving up. It's not a good feeling when all one wants to do is curl up in a ball and shut out the world.

While Carol's out golfing I took the opportunity to shave for the first time in eight days. I did a pretty good job all things considered. Using the electric razor around my incision was a bit tricky. When I was done I felt good about myself. For some reason it lifted my spirits. Who knows, maybe tonight I'll make a pass at Carol. . . WHOA! Easy boy. . . Not so fast. That could tear everything to shreds! Don't wanna start thinkin you're a fully functioning fellow just yet.

Today is September the 10th. Tomorrow I go to Salmon Arm to see my doctor and get my two week assessment. I know I'm healing quite well so there should be no problem. I also expect to start driving tomorrow. The end is in sight; I mean the end to this episode that has ruled my life for too long.

This afternoon I walked up town; about two miles return trip. The pain was the same as if I walked two or three blocks except I had to sit down and rest a couple of times. I took one Tylenol when I got home and had a short nap. I am so ready to move on.

I just got back from the doctor in Salmon Arm. Would you like to know what he told me. Good!

Firstly he said I was doing better than expected. Then he looked at his computer screen and said, "It's the best news possible. The cancer was in the best place possible and they're almost sure they got it all."

Sometimes you just get good news at the most opportune time and this was indeed an opportune time. When I asked him when he thought I could take up golf again he said, "Golf whenever you want. Do everything you did before."
Carol and I left his office with relief written all over our smiles. In a few days we are going to get our travel insurance for going to Arizona next month.

I took my doctor's advice and went golfing; even though everything in my right shoulder is still numb and weak. To my great surprise nothing hurt when I swung the club. The one thing I did notice however was I still have the same faults in my game. Every day I can feel the feelings coming back. Where the incision was will be a long time returning to normal. I'm okay with that.

Today is the eighteenth day since my surgery and the feeling is coming back into my right shoulder and around my right ear. However along the incision scar it is still quite numb. My shoulder gets sore and tired if I let it hang to long. Things are getting better.

Today is September 20th. I had a dream last night. I and two other people were walking along a path in nature. The child with us saw a beautifully coloured snake and ran towards it. Someone yelled "Copperhead" so I grabbed the child just as the snake left the ground and tried to bite the child. Then I saw another much larger snake which I assumed was the mother. It shot upward and bit me in my face. It was then when I woke up.

To me this was a good dream. It was the first one in a long time where the dream wasn't only about me. I was able to save a child from great pain and perhaps death. I am here and I am ready to get on with my life.

It's almost the end of September and I still have a lot of numbness in three areas. Some days I feel like an old man; I mean a old, old man. My aches and pains keep reminding me that I'm not the same as I used to be.

Maybe I'll just give up and hoist my pants up above my belt and wear outlandish clothes. That's the way I feel today. We leave for Arizona in two weeks. I hope my spirits are lifted when we depart.

After strong reflection about the way I feel inside, I know this bout of cancer has taken something out of me; or perhaps away from me. It's hard to put it into words but I seem to have lost some of my spirit. It may not show on the outside but something in my resolve is wounded.

Today is October 04th and our daughter phoned and told us our son in law had a heart attack. He's only forty seven years old. We're thankful it wasn't a big heart attack. It does make one think about the importance of living every day to the fullest.

The more I think about it the more I have convinced myself to enjoy the mysteries of life rather than the worries of death; keep every fibre of my being aware of the here and now. I will not sit idle and fret over death's inevitability. Cancer is only one way to die. Tomorrow I will throw myself into the waiting uncertainties of this world.

Seven

We are on our way to Yuma Arizona and I cannot tell you how elated I am. As of today we are in Hawthorne, Nevada with tire problems and because it's the week-end their two tire shops are closed. I do not call that a setback on the road of life; just on the road to Yuma. We'll enjoy our two or three days here and carry on. OH! My shoulder still hurts, especially after driving a couple of hours, but I know it is slowly healing. We have a great view out of our back window and the sun is shining. What more does a traveller need?

Today is October twenty third, twenty thirteen. We arrived here in Yuma yesterday. With everything behind me I look forward to enjoying this winter with Carol and good friends.

Part three

One

Here we go again. Today is June 04th, 2015 and I just found out I have to go to the Vernon hospital for a biopsy on my Prostate. The specialist said there is a lump on it and my PSA is high. I am at a loss for words to describe how that makes me feel; helpless, frustrated and scared.

Yesterday I thought everything was good because the Doctor took so long to set up the appointment that I figured everything was all right. Today I start living in fear of the unknown all over again. Tomorrow will come and the waiting will begin.

I know . . . I know, I have to keep a positive attitude and not get ahead of myself. WELL! I'm sorry, I expect the worst. My appointment is in a couple of weeks or so.

If the diagnosis is bad I don't know how I will be able to handle it. I am thinking long and hard on that.

This Sunday I golfed with Carol and a couple of friends. My right leg was killing me because of a degenerated disk in the bottom of my spine. I see the chiropractor tomorrow afternoon. I golfed okay but I was constantly thinking about what lies ahead. I'm not in a good place right now. Many thoughts run through my thinking. There is no one I can talk to so I must keep everything inside. I'm afraid if I start talking to Carol I will break down again. I am convinced I have prostate cancer and somehow must prepare myself for another battle.

Last night I laid awake thinking. The specialist knows I have cancer. Why would he tell me\ to see him two weeks after my biopsy so he can tell me the results? If it is negative why wouldn't they just phone me and tell me to have a good life.

I have a feeling this is going to be a short chapter. There's not much left to say. The call will come, I will go, tests will be performed and the specialist will deliver the news.

I had a short dream last night. A dark cloud floated above me as I walked. That was it.

I haven't put pen to paper for a few days. I've been in kind of a limbo waiting for the call. I feel good this afternoon. I took a puff of courage from the thin long dragon. I'm adjusting quite well.

My back problem is being resolved.

We had a good time golfing with friends today. I thought about death a few times. I'm trying to get my thoughts around the possibility . . . again! I have to go to my doctor tomorrow with new information about my condition. The specialist asked me if there was blood in my urine and at the time there was none. But for the last week there definitely is. It alarms me but he never told me what to do if I found blood in my urine.

Just in case you want to know, I'm still waiting for the call. Over ten days now. I find my spirits sagging under the weight of waiting.

I just wrote this poem.

Black poem

Death lives, tangled in the forest of darkness.
The black bloodhound stalks
the beasts in your dreaming.
The sun will be sucked from your sight
to blind you to the truth.
When evening retreats to darkness
beware of the ghosts of fear.
Sleep in the wilderness of terror
that haunts your forsaken ground.
The coming of morning's spears
will stab your eyes with golden light.
The high sun of noon will fill your dark soul with life.

There, that feels better.

    I'm still trying my best to figure everything out.
Unsafe thoughts seem to get in the way. OH! I know
things will unfold the way they must. And I'll shuffle
along from stage to stage. You'll see the hope in my
eyes, but you won't feel the fear in my heart.
.

I'm back.

    That last entry brought tears to my eyes. I still cry
easily. Now where was I. OH! Yes, death and its dark

secrets. I am half convinced it might be my time. I've yet to accept that. I have to stop now. This is not good for my thoughts.

Just in case you're wondering, I still haven't gotten the call. I still know I am important, but no more important than those ahead of me. I wonder if they'll give me a number and tell me to stand in line. I wonder how busy they are. It must be hard on the person who says, "You live . . . and you, you die." That's a heavy load to bear. Yet still, I'd rather be him than me. Will I see it in his eyes before he speaks? Will I be ready to accept whatever he says? I guess I'll have no choice.

I'll be back here tomorrow.

I just came back from a walk with my camera. I haven't done that, like, in forever. Even remembered how to operate the camera . . . sorta! I got a couple of nice pics. I like being alone. That's when I can do my more serious thinking; the thinking that really means something.

When I was twelve or thirteen me and my buddy would go over to the train tracks and watch the hobos.

When they left their camp to down town, we ransacked their camp. To this day I still feel bad about that.

Today is June 19ᵗʰ and I just found out I go for my biopsy in Vernon next week. It took me an hour and a half to compose myself after that. I wish I could control my emotions. I am expecting the worst because that's what I always get when it comes to this shit.

I got over the disappointment of starting all over with the worry of having cancer again. Got over it for now! It's time to put the blinders on and focus. Stiff upper lip and all that.

I cried today. Sometimes I get thinking the wrong thoughts. I hate being down.

What a great day at work today; upbeat and positive.

Tomorrow, who knows? We are celebrating our forty seventh wedding anniversary today, June 22, 2015. Who'd a thought she would stay with me that long? She has to be crazy in the head. I know how lucky I am.

I had my last treatment on my back today, for a while anyway.

Today is June the 24th. Tomorrow I go to Vernon. I left my job two hours early today; partly because of worry and I was caught up on the rough. Emotionally it's hard to focus in the right direction. Memories come back, I start thinking, remembering. I know it's not good for me. But that's the way it has to be, I guess.

Today I am ready to go to Vernon. I wish I knew what was in store for me.

Vernon went better than I had expected. Still, I'm happy that part is over.

When I looked into the mirror this morning I saw a seventy year old face staring back at me. I couldn't look at that person too long as he appeared to be somewhat older than that. Once again . . . it is what it is!

My dream last night took me to a place I often dream about. It's a small backwoods town with gravel streets. I have no idea where it is or what it represents. Maybe my dreams are preparing me for a journey to some place and want me to be familiar with it when I get there? There was a bus stop!

Last night I was feeling down. It all just came on me rather quickly. I didn't handle it very well. Today I'm feeling better. I wrote a poem after looking at this blank page before I used it.

This page is my temporary fate;
a place for my perfect truths.
This wide sheet of daring
a refuge for my leaping thoughts.
I shall assail it with a fury
from my melancholy heart.

There . . . I feel much better.
I came up with a sequel.

This page is an empty cell;
that anonymous place to sentence ones thoughts.
It is a worthy medium for truth.
What convenient accounting will it foretell?
I shall fatten its surface with honesty.

Two

I smoked a joint today. It was the first time in years. I
haven't been that relaxed in a long time. It definitely
mellowed me out.

I haven't been dreaming much lately. It kind of
bothers me because I usually have vivid dreams. What
does not dreaming, mean? I might goggle it.   I started
writing a poem for Carol for our fiftieth. It's only less
than three years away.

Today is July second and when I got up at four this
morning I looked out my window to see that my truck was
stolen during the night. I couldn't go to work. I called 9 1 1
and filed a police report and tried to contact ICBC.
But, guess what, ICBC is too busy to take my claim. I
had to go on line and do it. No personal contact just a
cold computer. When I was done on line it said they'd get
back to me in a couple of business days. I guess I'll just
sit here and twiddle my thumbs. Now I have no vehicle to

go to Salmon Arm and get my biopsy results. I am so stressed right now I don't know what I'm going to do.

I guess I know what's coming next. I had my biopsy, truck stolen and now I'm going to be told I have prostate cancer. Isn't that how it works? Everything comes in threes. In four days I get the news!

Today I am fine; yesterday not so much. I have never been so pissed off and bothered at a chain of events.

Three days to go before we get the results. We golfed with friends today and had a wonderful morning. We had lunch on the patio where we watched the golfers coming down eighteen. Carol had a alcoholic beverage which she seemed to enjoy. Today is a wonderful day. Tomorrow is a long way off.

Because I'm bored today I've decided to tell you something about myself. The day I joined the navy back in nineteen sixty three, I was excited for my future. I think that was the day I became a man. At least that's what I'd like to think.

I was going to join the army because my girl friend broke up with me and I thought I loved her. Isn't that what

I supposed to do; run off and seek adventure? Of course I ended up in the navy.

That also was the day I started my journey towards carol. I like to call it a chain of events.

Last night I took two Advile night-time pills t help me sleep. I never told Carol because the doctor said to take nothing other than extra strength Tylenol. I slept very well thank you!

Not a good morning. I had to leave the golf course after nine. Everything started coming down on me. I almost started to cry. That's when I feel my most helpless. When Carol gets home and wants to talk about it, that's when I'll cry; I always do when we talk about cancer. It's definitely beating me in the emotional department. It's time to suck it up and get back on the right track. I'll put the blinders on yet again, focus strong and steady towards my ultimate goal. You can cheer from the sidelines if you like. I could use the fans right now.

Now! Where was I? It has always amazed me how much better I feel after I write things down; a kind of sharing, if you will. I might just make through this day in a better mood. I'll let you know in due time.

I've come to the conclusion that it is time to mount the beast and hold on tight and yield nothing in my fight. If I can deal with his others, I should be able to deal with him. On days like this when the sun cannot find me I feel like gloom is stalking me.

What lies ahead is a dark mystery; I find that most frightening. My life does not need a disruption right now. Things were going good.

I started writing poetry this morning. I haven't done that for a while. Writing poetry centers me and my worries hide in the back ground. I wrote this poem thinking about old people who suffer.

Old timers

Mr. Brewster got lost because his life is hopeless and like a child he cries a lot.
Mom says he is beyond the repair of spare parts.

Sometimes he remembers why life saddens him
and it saddens him even more.
Last week he was a bird
but could not fly because a policeman
disrupted his take off.
Dad says Mr. Brewster was once a great pilot.
"but now he's just a bird in a cage"
I think he still has his dreams
and prefers them to giving up.
Some say he suffers from "old timers" disease.
Boy!
I wonder if God knows he's so discontented.

It always feels so good when I know how good a
poem can be! I am a majority of one when I say that.
I'm going to quit writing for the rest of the day. But I will
be here tomorrow, just like today and yesterday.

I've got two more days to go before I get the news. I'd
like to tell you I'm ready, but I'm not. My resolve is
dissipating. It's too hard to focus in the right direction.

Last night I slept well. I didn't tell Carol but I took two nighttime Advil. Today I got a rental car from ICBC. I was amazed how easy they made it. Tomorrow we go get the news.

Two

We just got back from seeing the specialist. All eight samples came back positive for cancer. It's time to put the blinders back on and get ready. A few more tests are need to determine how best to fight it. On the bright side, he said it was treatable. I found that rather encouraging.

I've been ready for this for some time now. I had made up my mind a ways back that I would have to fight again. I have the edge because I know a lot of what will happen going forward . . . bin there done that . . . I definitely have the edge.

Looks like Yuma is out of reach this winter. I'm disappointed for Carol. I'll find a way to make it up to her.

Today I'm reflecting back on yesterday. I was proud of
myself for holding it together. All I needed was an
answer; a simple yes or no. Now that the answer is yes
then it's time to get on with it. There is no time for tears.
I'll hold them in as long as it takes.
I just wrote this poem this morning.

Today I received the cold hard facts
which came in the form of an answer.
I just found out I have prostate cancer.

Today I learned I'm in for a fight
so I say bring it on, I'm ready.
My resolve is true and steady.

Tomorrow my new battle begins
all the cards are out on the table.
I'll struggle to the last if I'm able.

Tomorrow I fix my gaze to the future
where all my hope lies.
But, of course everyone dies.

Yesterday the waiting was killing me.

Today I'm damn well ready to fight.
Tomorrow I start to put things right.

Today is July the 10th, 2015. It has been at least two weeks since i remember having a dream. This has never happened before. I seldom go more than a few nights without dreaming. Now I must try to make sense of it. Is it a sign of what lies ahead; nothing?

Today I didn't want to be at work for some strange reason. I was in a down mood all morning long. It was a "Down beat day." Or a "Beat down day." All I know is it wasn't any fun.

Sometimes when I'm sad or a little down I write poetry. It centers me. It takes me in a new direction.

Oh what troubles I have seen
and what sorrow known.
Woe is me
with my heart of stone.

Now I feel better.

I took Carol to the golf club for supper; appies. When we got home we started talking about cancer and the possibilities of what might happen. When we read the side effects of some of the treatments I was concerned. It could affect everything from the taste of food to sex drive. Carol looked at me and said, "If there are certain things we cannot do anymore, we'll still have each other. I found that to be profound.

Today ICBC called me to settle the payment for my stolen truck. Of course it's way under what it actually is worth. But, we must live with it. I'm going to the Credit Union Thursday to see about another loan to get something newer. My fingers are crossed. I really didn't want to deal with this right now. More stress.

I received another doctor's appointment today. I know there's one more for sure in Vernon. Things are happening. Maybe it's a little too fast. Maybe they're trying to take me by surprise.

We are looking for another truck; much newer than the last one. I'm finally excited to start looking. It's a bummer to be truckless.

Today is Saturday; my first day off. We went golfing and I was sure I was going to have a great day. Boy! Was I wrong? For some unknown reason I couldn't concentrate on the shots. Frustration took over and it just got worse. I acted rather badly and am a little ashamed of my behaviour.

What once came so easily to me I now struggle to grasp. Fleeting memories come and go, but never when I need them. It starts with a brain fart; for no reason I can't remember a name I should remember.

Now I have to wing it. The other day I asked Carol what happened to old what's his name.

She snapped her head around and chortled, "Who the hell is "old what's his name?"

I say, "You know, he lived over by the bridge where that Lang boy jumped."

Her stare was breathtaking as she spoke, "OH! Are you thinking of old man Benson?"

Quickly I said yes. "Yes, whatever happened to him?"

"I haven't got a clue," she said as she turned her attention back to the book she was reading.

The funny thing is I never had a name in mind when I threw, "old what's his name out there." I figured it would go somewhere. And it did.

I am so happy that some things have turned around. I got the plates for my truck today. It should be ready to come home in a few days. I'm worried that someone else is going to steal it again. I'm looking into installing a anti theft device; an immobilizer. Only I will be able to start the truck. That would make me sleep better at night.

I think it's time to tell you something about myself that you may not know. Let me see . . . The first girl I ever kissed was fourteen and I was fifteen. My sister hazel set it up. When I kissed her on the lips goodnight . . . It was like kissing a two by four. To say I was disappointed would be a grave understatement. I don't know what I was expecting, but it wasn't that. I wondered if it was me, or her, or the both of us. It doesn't matter. I dumped her!

I was thinking at work today about something I shouldn't be thinking. I wonder why some people say things like, "OH! You'll be fine. My friend had it and he's fine."

What a stupid thing to say. Just shut up and say nothing. And the one, "You'll be fine, you beat it before."

Where's the comfort in that? I'll be what I'll be when the time comes.

I got was thinking this morning while riding the rough mower at work. How does one say good-bye? You know . . . that final good-bye. Will I be brave and tell a lie? Will there be a tear in my eye? I'd like to think I could be brave for my family. But somehow I think I'll cry when it comes my time to say good-bye.

Today is July 23rd. We found out today that I see the specialist at 12:45 tomorrow for our first test. I'm looking forward to having some good Chinese food while we're there.

Outside of the extreme discomfort of having my bladder inspected, I guess it was a good day. My bladder is in good shape; one down and a few more to go.

Today is Sunday and I golfed with my Wed. Men's team. We always play a friendly match for a few bucks. Today it was "Cry Wolf" and I skinned them for the second time in a row. They don't know my strategy because it's different than theirs. I'm sure they'll figure it out eventually. Of course I'll have a few more skins by then. Today I parred #12 by putting from well off the green. It was a great day. Tomorrow we head back to Salmon Arm.

I've had a lot of gas problems the last three weeks or so. The specialist said it was likely the frozen yogurt I have every night after supper. So Carol and I agreed that I would give up the yogurt for a week. She said, "If the farts go away during that time then it is the yogurt." I said, "If they persist then it's not the yogurt." I love my yogurt a lot. But I agreed. Every day she's not home I have my yogurt. What she doesn't know won't hurt her. As long as I keep farting she'll think it's not the yogurt. And besides what's a few farts anyway? Just keep that between you and me.

I just got back from my CT scan. That's another appointment over and done. Aug. 05th, here we come.

Carol's at ladies day today. I write poetry. Here is my last one.

A blanket smoothers the ground,
draping everything in a cloak of white.
My cold despair has been found
right here in plain sight.

Tomorrow I get my truck back. Fingers crossed!
Got the truck; went to the doctor today with five issues.
Gas, rash, blood spots on arms, flow max refill and feet cramping at night. Rash needs a cream for two weeks???

Everything was going along just fine. I was dealing with all my problems. Now we get a phone call from the Vernon hospital changing my appointment time back one week. That's another week I have to sit and wonder.

The woman that told me was so flustered she gave me the wrong times for my three appointments. She had to phone me back and it took a while to straighten it out. I don't know what her problem was but she said, "I'm looking at two screens and I got confused."

I'm a little ticked off right now. Damn! And I was feeling so good.

Today is Aug. 11th. Tomorrow we go to Vernon for more tests. I'm getting a little antsy. I try to keep calm and not think about it . . . BUT!

After that I have to wait another two weeks before I see the specialist and get the results. It'll Sept. before we get started with treatment.

Today I went to the doctor because I have no energy. Walking up the stairs is a chore. She said the cancer probably is what is doing it. Then she mentioned two other problems when she read the results of some of the tests. It didn't sound too good. I have a very bad feeling about what is to come. I must find a way to deal with it for my family. Without a doubt it will be the toughest challenge of my life.

Last night I had trouble getting to sleep. I spent some time thinking about my brother George and things that happened in our lives. Like the time when we were kids with bee bee guns playing cops and robbers. When he stuck his head out of the empty rain barrel I pulled the trigger and hit him square in the front tooth. Bull's eye! I guess it must be that time for me ... Remembering the past before I must grit my teeth and get ready for the future. If there is a future.

Today is Aug. 15th and it rained all night. I was awake for a lot of it. I had a few things to think about and sleep did not come easy. Carol's in a golf tournament today and tomorrow. I hope she thinks about golf today.

No matter how hard I try I simply cannot get what the doctor said about spots on my liver and lungs out of my mind. I am terribly concerned about the possibilities of what that means.

Today is Aug. 17th and I tried to golf nine holes this afternoon. I had no energy so I've decided to quit golf for a while. Also I'm thinking of quitting my job as I'm sure it contributes to my energy level. I don't want to quit but I think I must. Emotionally I'm having a tough time too. It's much tougher than the last two times.

Today I'm compiling a list of things I want to do before I pass away.
Say good bye to my wife and children with dignity. Tell them they are the reason I had such a great life. Don't be sad for me, I wouldn't have had it any other way.

Tell my brothers and sisters I love them.
Tell my friends I am grateful to have known them.

Go hiking one last time
Go hunting with my friends one last time
Go to sea one last time
Fish with my son one last time
Ride a motorcycle one last time
Hit one more home run one last time

Hug Carol
Hug Carol one last time.

This afternoon my doctor phoned me with some of the results. I have lesions in my liver my lungs and behind my heart. I have to go to Kelowna to see a specialist and let them biopsy it because they don't fit the prostate cancer scenario.

I quit my job just now.

Today is Aug. 18th and I decided to test my endurance by hiking up the Martha Creek trail. It's fairly steep and rocky and narrow. I climbed for forty minutes and then I was done. It took a while to gather my breath and start back down. I was rather light headed. I won't be doing that again. I fell twice. Hiking is out of the question! But the good news is, I tried and I'm damn proud of that. I discovered what I'm made of today and I'm really damn proud of that. Not to mention I was worried about meeting a bear on the trail. I'm happy I did what I did. I think today I strengthened my resolve. I guess I'll just stick to the kiddie's trails from now on.

I'm trying to fathom the thought of what's in store for me. I think the worst not having a clue at all. I smoked some marijuana this morning at 11:00 AM. I don't do it that early usually. It did make me feel better. It changed my focus.

I wrote this earlier this afternoon.

Spirits sometimes rise, and sometimes hammers fall.
No one knows when they're going to get the call.
Today is our day, another triumph for love and life.
I think I'll be just fine as long as you are my wife.

I dreamed about death last night. At least I think it was about death. There was a line of people walking up a steep hill carrying something but I couldn't tell what it was.

Today Carol's golfing with heather. I know I shouldn't say anything but today I smoked at 09:20. I know I shouldn't but as of right now I must. Don't ask me why because you know why. We both know why. Things are running rampant in my head and that seems to help me straighten them out. I make no apologies. I can tell you one thing for sure though . . . I didn't come all this far not to go all the way. Now where did I put those blinders?

I think it's time I tell you something about myself again.

I once had a friend OF Carol and I come on to me. It was when we were camping AT Raft River beach. I never told her about it. Her name was Tina. Cori was just a baby back then. I did the right thing and tactfully reclined her advances. And of course there's always the fear of getting caught.

Today I'm on a runaway train and I'm headed down the wrong track. Summer is flashing by as I careen alone. Try as I must I cannot stop it. My thoughts are like box cars shuttering along. What lies ahead only time will tell. What kinds of courage will I be able to muster; stiff upper lip and all that stuff?

My son came over for a visit around supper time. I haven't told him or his sister about my other problems with the lesions. Carol thinks I should tell them because they'll be mad when they find out. My view is that it's all part and parcel of prostate cancer. And besides, why get them worrying needlessly. And if they do get mad . . . Well! Boo Hoo!

Today is Sat. Aug. the 22nd. Carol is golfing after taking two days away from the game. I hope she does well. But if not there's always tomorrow.

As for myself . . . Well, let me see; I haven't shed a tear in three days. That is good. I baked raisin biscuits this morning and they are delicious. When I'm baking I must put all my focus on what I'm doing. I always don't get it perfect though. Like the recipe said to drop nine spoonfuls on an ungreased sheet. When I finished my drops I see only six drops on the sheet. So I used a round pan for the rest. The round one wouldn't fit on the same shelf as the square one so I put it on the shelf below it. Now do you see where I'm going with this? Yes! I burned the ones in the round pan. Lesson learned.

I feel poetic this afternoon. So if you don't mind I'd like to compose a verse. Wish me well.

I am the high priest of Marrakech
Waving my red flag to the breeze
Throughout this glorious day yet fresh
Lo it bought me to my knees.

What do you think.

Here it is only nine in the morning and I'm stoned; mostly because I don't want to go anywhere and have to talk about cancer. People don't realize how tough it is to handle it emotionally. Even as I write this I find myself starting to tear up.

I've been putting something off in my mind for quite a while now. I'd also appreciated if you wouldn't pre judge me when I make my next statement; suicide.

I attempted it once back in my twenties because of a girl and alcohol. This is obviously different. I do think about it often. I, unlike you probably, do not consider suicide as the coward's way out. Quite the contrary, it takes a brave individual to stand up and stare at all the avenues presented. It is simply one of the choices.

I never slept very well last night. I had chilli for supper two nights ago and then meat lover's pizza for supper last night. I don't know what I was thinking. I was up all night trying to pee. It was rather painful. Today i can feel the anxiety rising in me. Tomorrow is our big meeting on the video conference call with the specialist from

Kelowna. I don't know what's coming and it's killing me inside. I can't find any happy words today.

I just returned from a video conference with Dr. Luoma. He's a thoracic surgeon. It is the worst news possible. I have cancer in my lungs, my liver and my bones. Now I have to have another biopsy. This next one will be from my liver. He said Chemo therapy will be needed when the time comes to treat it. Now I sit and wait for another appointment. I still don't want our children to worry needlessly so for now Carol is just going to tell them that they found some spots and I have to go for another biopsy. If they get mad at me for not telling them up front then they can deal with it.

Three months ago I was an energetic happy golfer. Now I feel eighty years old with no energy and not much will to do anything. I think I know where this is going and I must find a way to deal with it. And I will.

Tomorrow I see Doctor Lavoie here at the hospital. I don't think he's going to tell me anything I don't already know.

Just got back from the doctor Lavoie and the news is not good. It could be a third kind of cancer. Another biopsy will be needed. Also there are lumps in my oesophagus. I think I'm pretty well fucked!

Just when I think I've got things figured out I kicked in the nuts. Oh! By the way that doesn't matter because everything down there is dead too. I know where this is going and so does Doctor Lavoie.

Today is Aug. 27th and we told our son and his family the bad news last night. I wasn't looking forward to it but we managed to get through it.

I had a dream two nights ago. I was running after the passenger train as it sped down the track. There was someone running behind me and I wondered why he couldn't keep up because I was seventy years old and I was catching it. I grabbed the grab iron and lifted myself up onto a step. Then my feet cramped up and I woke up.

I'm not sure what it means. Does it mean I've only got the past to look at?

This morning was the worst one ever. I'm glad carol is golfing. I couldn't hold it together. It all came flooding out. I sobbed long and loud and angry. I hope all theses tears are leading me somewhere. I feel so helpless when I cry.

I had a long chat with Jane and for the first time talked about death. I have to find a way to accept it. I can tell you that right now I am as terrified right now as I have ever been or ever will be. It's squeezing my heart. The emotional pain is almost unbearable. I have to get my shit together before carol comes home. She doesn't need to know. I'm sure she has her own problems and must find her way to deal with them. We will have that serious talk . . . just not ready yet.

I had a small victory this afternoon but I don't want to talk about it just now. I think I've got myself together. Carol should be home anytime.

This morning we golfed nine holes. I took a cart. It was really frustrating but the fresh air was good. I did manage two pars near the end. I threw my clubs in the back seat of the truck.

We went to Todd's this afternoon and had a nice Barbeque with Cori and Jeff and Paige and Connor and Jamie. Not one tear was shed. Not sure what to make of that?

Today is Aug. 31st and it rained all night and is pouring down now. It could not be more depressing. Sitting and waiting again is not fun.

I managed to get two appointments today; one for my throat here in Revelstoke on the 9th with Dr Weismann. Then the next day in Salmon Arm for a liver biopsy. Things are starting to move. I guess it's time to hold on.

I cried for the first time in two days today. After getting the appointments I cried. I guess that's what makes it real. I tried to keep it out of my mind.

We finally made the decision to house sit this winter for Dawn and Gary. At least that's one thing settled. I know it will be for the best.

I have trouble hugging Carol. I can only hug her for a few seconds at a time. Any longer and my emotions boil to the surface. I hate crying!

We went to my doctor today. I even cried in his office. As hard as I tried not too I could not hold back the tears. When that word is spoken to me I cannot handle it.
The fear that lies ahead of me is emotionally draining me.

Today Carol is finally golfing. I hope she has a good round. Me, I'm bored.

I thought I had no more appointments until next Wed. But this afternoon the phone rings and tells me to come up to the hospital for blood samples and an EKG. So I went and had that done. It's hard trying to keep track of everything going on.

Today is September the forth. This morning I've decided it's time to do my last will and testament. I don't have much but it still should be in order. I want to make this as easy on Carol as I can. I have a life insurance policy that should help a bit.

I've also starting thinking about where I would like my ashes spread. Probably seventeen mile but we'll get to that later.

I got a call today from Salmon arm hospital telling me I have another scan to do when i get there next Thursday. So that's two scans, one a biopsy scan, one a CT scan and a liver biopsy. Now we have to be there early.

Today Carol's in the Labour Day golf tournament. Me, I'm still trying to fathom a few things. I had a long night Last night. I couldn't control my mind. I smoked at ten thirty this morning. From now on I'm going to do what I'm going to do; right or wrong?

I want to leave this earth without regret for things I should or shouldn't have done. I've always been able to take what was thrown at me. I never had many complaints because I knew that life was life so you better take it as it comes. But I must tell you I hadn't bargained for this.

Carol helps keep me on course but I can't talk to her about it or I start with the crying all over again. I'm sure she knows how much i need her. It's going to take all the courage we can muster from here on. When they finally give me the bad news; I'll have to live every second of the time I have left. Nothing lasts forever.

Today is Sunday. Carol's golfing. This morning for some reason I feel so alone; like I'm stranded somewhere with no way of escape. And the bad thing is I don't know how to deal with it. My fear is that I'll have a nervous breakdown when I need my strength the most. I'm working on it but the progress is not there.

I just got back from a drive up to the cabin up the Big Bend Highway. I thought It would lift my spirits but there are two families from merit there who think they own the place. Now I wish I hadn't gone. But, it might be the last chance I had to go. Cross that off my list.

After I got home I smoked and made the bold decision to let it all out. I spend so much time and effort to keep everything in I just had to let it all out. For some reason I couldn't cry. Nothing happened . . . no tears, I don't get it. When Carol comes home and even hints at that word I bawl like a wounded calf.

I guess now that I'm stoned I might as well tell you something about myself.

When I was in the navy and at sea I was put in charge of serving and looking after the non commissioned officers mess. It was my duty to clean the place up and get it ready for breakfast the next morning. One night I came back a wee bit drunk and when i went to clean the mess it was an absolute disaster. It was a pig pen. So I locked the door and went to bed. Needless to say the next morning I was rudely awoken and ordered to the mess. I cleaned it and served breakfast. I was put up on charge for derelict of duty.

When the captain read the charges to me and asked me if I had anything to say in my defence, I responded thusly; "Sir, when I came back to the ship last night I went to the mess to get it ready. I could not believe how filthy they had gotten it. It looked like there was a food fight or something. That's when I made the decision; if they want to live like pigs."

The Captain bought it when he said, "I agree, you're free to go. But the only reason I say that is because when you were placed there you were to assist them, it was not your duty to do everything for them."

That's the same Captain who would later remind me that my charge sheet was full . . . front and back. God! I must have loved being in trouble back then. But now it doesn't seem like it was any trouble. What a great memory. Man I feel good.

When Carol got home from golf this evening I was going to tell her about my drive up to the cabin. But when I started thinking about it I got choked up and couldn't do it. I guess that's what love does to a man in my predicament. It might even be a good thing. I don't know.

When the stars all disappear
and death has taken my breath,
what last hurdle will I fear?
before I meet my death.

This morning is a downer. I guess because tomorrow is coming. I smoked at 09:00 and Carol is home. I know she understands. Not sure she approves though. Another rainy day of sitting and waiting.

I can't have anything to drink or eat after midnight tonight. It will be twelve or more hours without sustenance. I'm going to talk Carol into taking me out Friday night to Zalas. After all she did win the fifty, fifty pot at the Labour Day tournament. Three hundred and twenty dollars.

Dr. Wiseman scoped my Oesophagus and said the inside is good. But there is an ulcer pushing against it and its most like cancerous. They will know in a few days. If it is it can't be removed. He said they can control it . . . Whatever that means. He says I'm a work in progress.

Today should be my last biopsy????? We leave in five minutes. For some reason I'm optimistic and ready to do this. Everything went fine with the biopsy. Now I wait again.

Today I just t=received a call from Vernon to go see Dr Humphries next Thursday for a one hour appointment. That seems like a rather long appointment. Not sure if that's good or bad. Of course you know what I think. I just hope this is not going to be too hard on Carol and the kids. I've known for some time now

what is coming. I can feel it inside of me. I try to be
optimistic.

There's a storm brewing in front of me,
    waiting patiently for me to take flight.
    But I boldly and strongly disagree,
    this time I will win the fight.

There . . .
That's optimistic!

Today Carol is golfing. Me, well you know what I'm
doing. I'm still struggling with it all. I know I have to make
out my last will. I guess I'll wait until after next Thursday.
Todd came over and watched the Jays last night. It was
good for me. And Dawn and Gary came for a while.
Carol made finger food.
    I just finished goggling "Why do we cry? It is a long
and complicated explanation. I found out there is nothing
I can do to stop crying when my emotions overwhelm me .
. . Nothing!
    I've been trying to figure out where my head is for
the last few weeks. I'm never completely in the presence.
Sometimes I spend too much time looking into that other

place. It's not a good feeling. I just wish I could find something to be happy with, anything at all. I know there are people out there who know exactly what I'm talking about, but sadly many of them have passed on.

This afternoon I'm in a pensive mood. I wonder how many people actually get to know what it's like to be so alone with your thoughts and fears. Of course it's indescribable, like so much of this business. If there is a way to reason it out I sure can't find it. I guess I'll just keep carrying on.

Today is Sunday and Carol and I went and golfed nine. I took a cart and am glad I went. I still find it very difficult to have someone come and talk to me. Don't ask me why? It's going to be a rough couple of days leading up to Thursday. Not sure how I'm going to handle it.

Carol and I just have a discussion about how she screwed up the Yorkshire pudding the last two times she tried to make it. She had excuses; like it's the oven, it doesn't cook the same on both sides. The truth is she doesn't want to cook anymore. She knows it and I know it. So what does old big mouth do; I volunteer to make it the next time. I guess my roast beef eating days are over because I sure as hell am not making Yorkshire pudding.

Today is Monday the fourteenth of September. I slept very well last night, but after i got up the tension started rising in me. It drained me of my energy. I couldn't wait to take Carol to the golf course and get home and smoke. I can feel the tension easing away as I type. I don't know how I will be able to handle this coming Thursday.

I would love to experience the comfort of a worry free day. It's been so long I can't remember the last time that happened. This god-damn thing is consuming me. It's killing me before we get a chance to fight.

We went out for wings tonight at the Rockford with Dawn and Gary. I was glad I went. I still don't want to talk to others about my problem but it seems every time we go out I have to. We had a great time.

This morning I smoked at 08:30 and had my worst breakdown so far. This fucking cancer is killing me. Carol wants me to talk to someone. What can someone tell me if they haven't experienced what I'm going through? If I could dispose of myself right now I would. Thank God Carol's stronger than I am. Without her none of this would matter.

Yesterday's melt down is behind me. Today is going rather well. I took Carol golfing at 10:00. Tomorrow is probably the biggest day of my life; do I live or do I die? It's all in Dr Humphrey's hands. Whatever his decision is I must find a way to handle it.

Well! That didn't go as planned. We just got back from the Oncologist in Vernon where I thought I would get some answers; like what kind of cancer is this new one, what kind of treatment will it take and when do we start. NO! NO! NO! They don't know yet. They think it might be from the Acinar cell Carcinoma and it got into my blood stream. I have to get an appointment with another specialist in Kelowna and have another CT scan. Of course that will take a week to ten days to get that one. This is finally giving me hope. The way I see it is if they keep putting it off I may just die of old age.

Today is September the 18th. It's 05:00 am and I feel good. I have one month to wait so I might as well relax and get on with it. I am going to golf today . . . if it stops raining? Today was my best day in over two months. We golfed with Gary and I was relaxed all day. I guess a time-out is good.

Today it rained all day. Boring, boring, and boring!

Today is Sept. 20th and this morning is my worst morning. I cannot shake this depression. I know Carol is extremely disappointed with me and so she should be. The rain hasn't stopped for three days and it only adds to everything. I cannot take another day like today. There are no words to tell you the depth of my despair. I don't know what brought it on or why it happened but I have never experienced anything like it before. I hope it is behind me.

Today Carol and I went golfing. She was going to do nine with me and then join the girls for eighteen. I ran out of stamina and had to quit on #5.

I just found out this afternoon an interesting fact. The average age of a human at death is seventy years old. I fit the profile perfectly. So what's my problem?

Today when I was shopping at Coopers a railroader I used to know came up to me. I can't remember his name right now. He said, "I know just how you feel".

I asked him what kind of cancer he had.

Turns out he's never had cancer . . . He just KNOWS how I feel. What kind of asshole talks like that? That's the last thing I want or need to hear! Sometimes a person will just talk because they feel the need to respond, even though they don't know what to say. I guess I could help them by telling them what I'm OK talking about and what I'm not. I could also tell them that I only need them to listen to me, and that I don't need them to say anything other than that they care and are there for me, but unfortunately that's not me. Sometimes I wish it was but it's just not.

Tomorrow I'm going to golf my last men's day and my last this year. My strength is low but I have a good feeling. Concentration is the key! Wish me luck.

This morning while I was drying the dishes I dropped another one smashing it all over the place. It was a dinner plate. A couple of weeks ago I did the same to a saucer. I don't know if it's because I'm not paying attention or something else. And now I can't find the extra lighters I bought. Haven't got a clue where I put them. Carol probably knows. Just four more hours and I'll be golfing. . . Well! Maybe I'll just be hitting a ball.

I just found my lighters and they were right where I had put them.

Once I told Neil about my cancer I received an e-mail from him offering to come for a visit with my other buddy Danny.

Hi again,

You seem to have a problem delivering good news. Are you feeling ok and able to do your day to day activities like golfing or chasing Carol around the house?

Are you taking any medications until the doctors figure things out? I Talked to Danny after your e mail and we thought it would be a good idea to ask you if we could come and see you for a little support and to cover up our reasons for not stopping to see you this summer! This decision would of course be yours and we would stay at the Sandman for one night or possibly two. If we were to come it would be early next week, but I would have to check with Danny first. Give me a heads up on what you think.

Neil

I was so overcome with emotion that they thought that much of me. It brings tears to my eyes as I type. I Know I couldn't handle it so I had to turn them down. I wish I could but I know I can't.

This afternoon I hugged Carol and I Still couldn't do it without tearing up. The longer I hold her, the harder it is on me.

Today is Sunday the 27th. For some strange reason Carol told me this morning that my lungs were fine. She saw the same slides I saw and she knows there's cancer in them. I don't get it?

Up and until now I thought I was doing quite well. I accommodated her for rides without failure and I try to support her as best I can. I'm not stupid; I know I can't get through this without her. I don't expect her to understand what I'm going through because she can't. I hope things don't go downhill from here.

I left this message on the lap top for her to read because if I try to say the words to her I know I'll cry.

Carol

I'm sorry. I know this is not fair for you. I wish there was something I could say but there isn't. I'm trying the best I know how.

My tasted buds over the last while have abandoned me. Anything cooked has very little flavour. Sweets still taste fairly good. It's hard to describe but most food taste nothing like it should. I have to eat so I eat and get through it. I guess it's just another roadblock I must figure out. On the other side my eye problems seem to be getting a bit better.

This morning I went to Southside and got two bags of kitty litter for when we store the fifth wheel for the winter. It was all I could do to pack them to the truck and get them into the front seat. Why am I so zapped of strength? I hope I don't have to take them back.

My tasted buds are done. Nothing taste like it should. And textures are different. Sweets aren't too bad. I'll try to keep my mouth shut and just eat what I can.

Today is Tuesday the 29th. Carol's golfing ladies day so i set up an appointment to see a Notary Public to make out my will. It was tougher than I thought it would be. I made Carol and Gary my decision maker in case i can't. I hope Gary agrees. We have to go sign the papers next week sometime.

I feel like a half a person walking around town. It's like I'm in a fog and only half there. It's not a good feeling. I don't know how I come across to others.

It is a tough morning this morning. Had to go to the optometrist to find out my eye infection is from herpes. She said from my cold sores. Of course I cried. Then we had to take the truck to the Ford dealer because it had trouble starting. It's just one thing after another. The optometrist said my eye should get better in a day or two. I hope so because it is very irritating. It's time to suck it up again and get back on track.

My brother Bert is coming for a visit today. It'll be good to see him. We had a great visit. Thanks Bert.

This morning I had a bad melt down. Thank god Carol's stronger than me. It took her a while but she straightened me out. I'm trying to get back on course.
This afternoon I'm back on track. We went for two walks and I feel good again.

This morning we got up at 05:00. I smoked at 05:30 to try and relax. It seems to be working. The optometrist says my eye is almost healed. It feels great again; a rather boring day for Carol what with all the rain. I phoned Bro. Geo. I had a visit this morning from Ron Cameron. We got caught up on a few things. I'm looking forward to tomorrow.

Carol started moving stuff into the house today. I could feel her reluctance to getting it done. She did quite a bit. I'm doing all my stuff tomorrow when she's golfing. That way there will be no arguments.

Carol's golfing her last ladies day today. I hope she has a good game. Me . . . I've been thinking again. I know I have one foot in the grave; I've known it for a month or more now. I just want to get on with what might be left. I'm hoping for at least another eight months. I guess time will tell.

Today is Monday the fifth of Oct. I got my truck back from the Ford dealer this afternoon. There was no issue with it. That made me so happy. I was thinking the worst again.

I just got back from my doctor. He sent me straight to the hospital to have my blood platelets checked. I went and had it done . . . Again. Jesus Christ when does it stop?

I try not to view it as a setback, but it doesn't appear to be advancing anything. How much blood do they need? Doctor Jarmula phoned to tell me that my potassium level is low and I have to go to the drug store first thing in the morning and get another prescription. More pills to take.

Carol's still moving stuff across to the house. I think she's into it now. I'll just stay out of the way and keep my mouth shut.

Today is October 8th. We move today. I couldn't make it to the end of the sidewalk this morning. I am getting even weaker than before. I won't say anything because it will just add to the stress.

We are moved into the house. It isn't too bad. I love the way Dawn and Gary take everything in stride. Me; I'll just go with the flow. Carol did an awesome job.

Went to the optometrist today and my eye is ninety percent cured. She sent me back to the doctor so went to him to get pills to clear up cold sores. It took forever to see him. The stress was almost unbearable. The fifth wheel is ready to go tomorrow.

Today is Sat. My rig is gone. I'll try to give Carol her space today.

Today is Thanksgiving Day. At ten this morning I started getting severe pains in my lower abdominal. I was taken to the hospital and rushed me to the hospital in Vernon by ambulance. A CT scan confirmed that my cancer was terminal. I had two choices; have a very risky operation that I probably would not survive. So I chose what's behind door # 2 ... Death.

Okay. I'm ready for that. I'm currently in the hospital in Revelstoke and have family and friends. We don't know how long it will be but that's okay too. I cannot thank all the specialists and doctors and nurse for their dedication to their duties. I am the luckiest person for my life to end surrounded by family and friends.
Whoever reads this I want to tell what I've written was written as honestly as I could.

I'm just glad that I got to finish it.